PRE- AND POSTOPERATIVE CARE OF THE CATARACT PATIENT

PAUL C. AJAMIAN, O.D., FAAO

Butterworth–Heinemann
Boston   London   Oxford   Singapore
Sydney   Toronto   Wellington

Library of Congress Cataloging-in-Publication Data

Ajamian, Paul C.
 Pre- and postoperative care of the cataract patient / Paul C. Ajamian.
  p.   cm.
 Includes bibliographical references and index.
 ISBN 0-7506-9073-9 (: alk. paper)
 1. Cataract—Surgery.   I. Title.
 [DNLM: 1. Cataract Extraction.   2. Postoperative Care.
 3. Preoperative Care.   WW 260 A312p]
 RE451.A42   1993
 617.7'42—dc20
 DNLM/DLC
 for Library of Congress   92-16080
                                                    CIP

British Library Cataloguing-in-Publication Data.

A catalogue record for this book is available from the British Library.

Butterworth–Heinemann
80 Montvale Avenue
Stoneham, MA 02180

10 9 8 7 6 5 4 3 2 1

Printed in the United States of America

This book is dedicated to my wife, Susan, and to my parents, Charlie and Nectar, for their unfailing love and support, and to the memory of my dear friend, Dr. Bill Barrett.

CONTENTS

PREFACE

Optometry's role in the management of the cataract patient has changed dramatically over the past decade. With expanded scope of practice laws and enhanced clinical education, doctors of optometry are actively involved in diagnosing and monitoring cataracts and in deciding (along with the patient) when surgery should be performed. Once a surgical referral is made, the optometrist's involvement with the patient's care is no longer over. More and more optometrists are now an integral part of the patient's postoperative care. This may begin as early as one week or as late as three to six months after surgery. The degree of involvement is dependent on many things, including the confidence of the surgeon in the optometrist's skills and in that surgeon's own technical ability and complication rate. For true co-management to occur, the surgeon must give up that part of the global surgical fee that covers postoperative care, something that a dwindling number of surgeons are willing to do in an era of declining reimbursement.

This text was written with these rather dramatic changes in mind. It is designed to assist practitioners and students alike by presenting the most common clinical approaches to the management of pre- and postoperative cataract patients. Chapter 4 reviews current surgical procedures in order to assist doctors in recognizing state-of-the-art versus mediocre results.

Chapter 7 deals with regulatory and reimbursement issues. It also provides an overview of co-managed care between the doctor of optometry and the surgeon, an eye-care model on which our practice and this text are based.

This book is written as a practical clinical guide to the situations most commonly encountered by the private practitioner, not as an exhaustive literature review laden with studies and statistics. I hope you enjoy it.

ACKNOWLEDGMENTS

I am indebted to a number of people who helped make this book possible. I would like to thank my close friend and colleague, Dr. Robert Pinkert, who was a major contributor to Chapter 1 and who also reviewed the entire text. Dr. Jim Thimons and Dr. Tony Cavallerano also spent many thoughtful hours reviewing the manuscript, and I am most grateful for their expertise. Special thanks also go to Drs. John Amos and Murray Fingeret, who shared their experiences as accomplished optometric authors and encouraged me from start to finish.

In addition, I gratefully acknowledge the role my staff played in the completion of this book—the many hours of transcribing and editing by Barb Graham, photographic assistance by Mike Packwood, C.R.A., and Medicare/insurance expertise and the constant support of Darlene Bradley.

I would also like to thank the editorial and production staff at Butterworth–Heinemann, especially Barbara Murphy for her encouragement and kindness.

Finally, special thanks go to those individuals without whom there might never have been a need for a text such as this: to William Wallace, O.D., for his role as one of the pioneers of the co-management concept and to the directors of the other co-management centers across the country, each of whom has helped elevate the profession of optometry to new heights.

Finally my deep gratitude to Ralph C. DiIorio, M.D., for his surgical expertise, his review of Chapter 4, and most of all for his long-standing commitment to doctors of optometry in Georgia and around the nation. He has always believed that optometrists should be integrally involved in the management of postoperative cataract patients and in all aspects of eye care. He had the courage to stand up for these beliefs long before co-management was accepted by his colleagues. For this, the profession of optometry will always be indebted to him.

1

Overview of Cataracts

□

■
ANATOMY AND PHYSIOLOGY OF THE CRYSTALLINE LENS

The crystalline lens is a unique, optically clear organ located behind the iris, bounded anteriorly by the aqueous and posteriorly by the vitreous. The lens is held in place by zonular fibers that are anchored in the ciliary processes and attach to the lens equator. These zonules act in conjunction with ciliary muscle contraction to change the shape and refractive power of the lens during the process known as *accommodation*. The lens supplies approximately one-third of the refractive power of the human eye.

The lens is covered by the capsule, an elastic basement membrane that serves to maintain its structural integrity. Beneath the anterior lens capsule is the epithelium, a single layer of cuboidal cells that multiply throughout life. These cells migrate to the equator where they elongate into lens fibers. As new fibers form beneath the anterior and posterior capsule, older fibers are displaced toward the center of the lens. This process continues throughout life, resulting in a gradual increase in the size of the lens. This central lens core is known as the *nucleus*. The area between the nucleus and the anterior or posterior capsule is called the *cortex* (Figure 1.1).

The transparent nature of the crystalline lens depends on both physical and chemical factors. The arrangement of the lens fibers, the relatively dehydrated state of the lens (65 percent water), and the presence of a high concentration of protein (34 percent) all contribute to optical clarity. Glucose metabolism and the production of ATP provide energy to maintain this transparent state and to allow for cell growth.

■
CATARACT FORMATION

A *cataract* is an opacity of the crystalline lens, either focal or diffuse. Some clinicians reserve the term for those opacities that affect visual acuity. Others

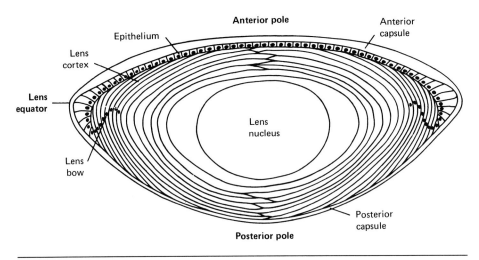

Figure 1.1   Diagrammatic section through the human lens, showing lens epithelial cells migrating to the equator where they elongate into lens fibers. (Reproduced with permission of the publisher from Records R. Physiology of the Human Eye and Visual System. Hagerstown, Md.: Harper & Row Publishers, 1979.)

make the diagnosis at the first sign of lenticular yellowing. There are no definitive guidelines as to when to label a lens opacity a cataract, but the individual's visual acuity level and emotional makeup should play a role in the decision.

The vast majority of cataracts are age-related, but there are other etiologies (Table 1.1). Several characteristic changes take place in the human lens with age:

• The lens enlarges as new fibers are produced.
• The older fibers become compacted toward the center of the lens (sclerosis).
• A yellow-brown pigment accumulates.
• Water enters the lens cortex.

The physical changes of fiber growth, intake of water, and chemical alterations of lens protein, enzyme, and electrolyte levels all contribute to lens opacification. The process is still not completely understood.

It is also believed that ultraviolet light not absorbed by the cornea plays a role in the progressive pigmentation of lens protein. There is mounting evidence that supports an association between long-term exposure to ultraviolet light and the formation of cataracts.

Congenital	Systemic disease related
Remnants of the tunica vasculosa lentis	Diabetes
Zonular	Hypoparathyroidism (hypocalcemia)
Nuclear	Metabolic storage disease
Polar	Myotonic dystrophy
Total	Atopic dermatitis
Age-related	**Drug-induced**
Nuclear	Steroids
Cortical	Phenothiazines
Posterior subcapsular	Miotics
Secondary	**Traumatic**
Uveitis	Blunt
Hereditary retinal disorders	Penetrating
Glaucoma	Radiation
Retinal detachment	Electric shock
Degenerative myopia	

Table 1.1   Classification of Cataracts

■ TYPES OF CATARACTS

☐ Congenital Cataracts

Congenital cataracts are those that arise in utero or during early infancy and development. The opacities are often small enough that they do not interfere with vision, but they may also be axial and dense enough to cause reduced acuity and possible amblyopia.

The cause of congenital cataracts is often unknown. Those causes that can be identified include:

- Maternal drug use or abuse
- Exposure to radiation during pregnancy
- Maternal malnutrition
- Metabolic disease (diabetes, galactosemia)
- Maternal or fetal infection (rubella)

Congenital cataracts are categorized by their location within or around the lens as is described below.

REMNANTS OF THE TUNICA VASCULOSA LENTIS

Persistence of the fetal network of vessels (the tunica vasculosa lentis) that surrounds the lens during development leads to characteristic opacities. Fortunately these rarely affect vision and include:

Persistent pupillary membranes. Seen as fine threads attached to the iris collarette or anterior lens capsule, these may atrophy and disappear with age.

Epicapsular stars. Pigmented spots found coalesced on the anterior lens capsule. Although quite striking in appearance when they are densely packed, they do not affect visual acuity (Figure 1.2).

Mittendorf's dot. A white dot just nasal to the visual axis on the posterior capsule. It represents the site of attachment of the hyaloid artery during embryonic development and also has no effect on visual acuity.

ZONULAR (LAMELLAR) CATARACT

Intermittent disturbances of the developing lens fibers result in *zonular or lamellar* opacities. The extent of the cataract depends on the duration of exposure to the disruptive stimulus. The outer portion of the fetal nucleus or the inner portion of the adult nucleus is most often affected. These opacities may be made of numerous fine white dots, or they may be solid in appearance (Figure 1.3). This central opacity may be associated with radial spokelike opacities called *riders*. Vision is often severely affected.

NUCLEAR

Injury to the embryonic or fetal nucleus during the first trimester can give rise to nuclear opacities. These may interfere with vision, depending on their size and density. The *pulverulent cataract* is a dominantly inherited bilateral opacity that appears as a ball of pinpoint white dots in the central nucleus (Figure 1.4).

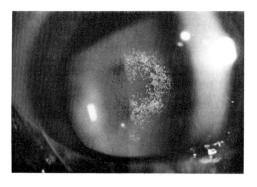

Figure 1.2
Epicapsular stars on the anterior lens capsule.

Figure 1.3
Zonular cataract with riders.

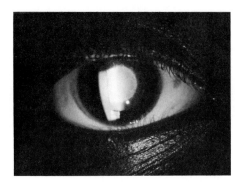

POLAR CATARACTS

Opacification of the subcapsular lens cortex can lead to anterior or posterior *polar cataracts*. These opacities may be hereditary, or they might be the result of fetal inflammation. Commonly disk-shaped, these opacities are often bilateral, symmetrical, and of variable size. Occasionally an anterior polar cataract will extend forward into the anterior chamber, termed a *pyramidal cataract*. Posterior polar opacities are more likely to cause vision loss because of their location. These cataracts are generally non-progressive throughout life.

TOTAL OR SUBTOTAL CATARACT

Rarely, primary lens cells will fail to grow due to a severe disturbance during the developmental period. The lens nucleus may be entirely absent, which gives rise to a white mass representing degenerated cortex. This is known as a *total* or *subtotal cataract*.

CORONARY OR CERULEAN CATARACT

Congenital opacities scattered throughout the lens cortex are relatively common. They may present as white punctate dots known as *coronary cataracts* (Figure

Figure 1.4
Pulverulent cataract.

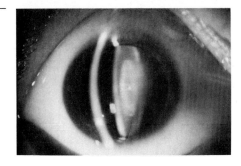

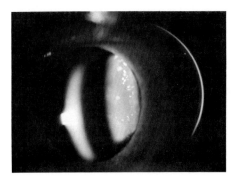

Figure 1.5
Coronary cataract representing congenital opacities of the lens cortex.

1.5) or take on a bluish hue, referred to as *cerulean* or *blue-dot cataracts*. They are generally non-progressive and cause no patient symptoms.

☐ Age-related Cataracts

Cataracts that appear in or after the third to fourth decade of life are referred to as *age-related* or *senescent*. A majority of individuals over the age of 60 will show some yellowing or loss of transparency of the lens, which rarely interferes with visual acuity early on. With time, denser opacities may develop that affect the nucleus, cortex, posterior subcapsular zone, or in many cases, a combination thereof.

NUCLEAR SCLEROSIS

The normal human lens nucleus becomes harder or more *sclerotic* with age. This condition is accompanied by a color change, either yellow, amber, brown, or milky white. The sclerosis creates a higher index of refraction, often resulting in a gradual and sometimes significant myopic shift. This myopic shift is responsible for the phenomenon known as *second sight*, which allows patients to read without glasses for the first time since before presbyopia. Some patients retain excellent distance acuity for a period of time with incremental prescription changes.*

Often the myopic shift is unequal between eyes, creating significant anisometropia. Unequal adds or slab-off prism may become necessary. Eventually the anisometropia itself may become a compelling reason to recommend surgery even in the presence of relatively good acuity. Monocular diplopia, ghost images, and a difficult endpoint during refraction may also be characteristic of nuclear sclerosis (NS).

---

*When adding minus power to a distance prescription, be prepared to compensate by adding more plus at near. Leave the patient with the equivalent near prescription they were accustomed to before the distance change.

Figure 1.6
Retroillumination of cortical water
vacuoles and peripheral spokes.

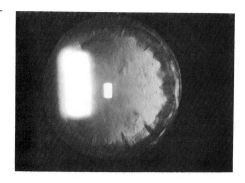

An importance distinction should be made between typical brunescent NS (Plate 1) and *milky* NS (Plate 2). The clinical appearance of milky NS has been described in a variety of ways, including a small central zone of haziness, mother-of-pearl, or opalescence of the nucleus. Frequently there is a lucid interval surrounding the central opacity, giving the appearance of a lens within a lens.

CORTICAL CATARACT

Cortical cataracts result from fluid intake into the cortex, leading to separation and degeneration of lens fibers. Clinically this takes the form of vacuoles, dots, water clefts, or peripheral spokes. Water vacuoles are best seen with retroillumination using the red reflex of the fundus (Figure 1.6). These vacuoles and punctate cortical opacities rarely cause visual acuity loss unless they become coalesced on the visual axis. Water clefts are clear, radially oriented changes that represent lens fiber separation. Opacification of these clefts leads to formation of grey-white cortical spokes, often extending toward the visual axis (Figure 1.7). Cortical spoking is seen anteriorly more frequently than it is seen posteriorly and

Figure 1.7
Cortical spokes extending toward the
visual axis.

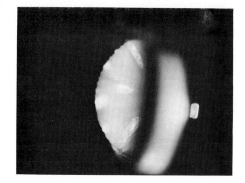

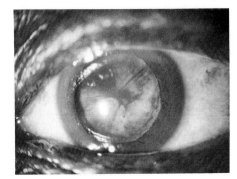

Figure 1.8
Wedge-shaped cortical opacification commonly affects the inferior temporal and inferior nasal quadrants.

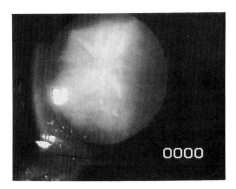

Figure 1.9
A mature white cortical cataract.

often takes the form of triangular wedges in the inferonasal or temporal quadrants (Figure 1.8).

With age, water continues to collect in the cortex. This intumescence may lead to shallowing of the anterior chamber and a secondary risk of angle closure glaucoma in predisposed eyes. The cortex can become so liquified that the lens becomes completely white (Figure 1.9). In rare cases, the nucleus sinks inferiorly within the liquified cortex, resulting in a *Morgagnian cataract* (Plate 3).

Posterior Subcapsular Cataract

Posterior subcapsular cataracts (PSCs), a subgroup of cortical cataracts, are a very common form of age-related lens opacity. These changes seem to affect younger patients (40s and 50s) as well and can be very debilitating because of their frequently central location. Progression is often more rapid than with cortical or nuclear changes. For these reasons, earlier surgical intervention may be required. Before a diagnosis of age-related PSC cataract is made, it is important to rule out:

Figure 1.10
PSC as viewed in retroillumination.

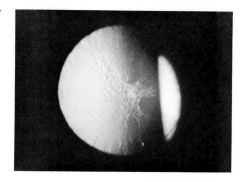

- Chronic topical or systemic steroid use
- Chronic uveitis
- Retinitis pigmentosa
- Systemic disease

Clinically, early PSCs are best visualized by retroillumination using the red fundus reflex (Figure 1.10). This can be accomplished with the direct ophthalmoscope or the slit lamp biomicroscope. With direct illumination, the opacity may appear as a granular whitish plaque (Figure 1.11). PSCs typically involve the visual axis but can also be seen peripherally affecting one or more quadrants.

Although small in size, the PSC may have a surprising effect on visual acuity. It is frequently responsible for symptoms early in the course of the disease process. The proximity of the cataract to the nodal point of the visual system explains this dramatic effect on vision. Patients frequently complain of decreased vision while reading, problems with bright sunlight, and difficulty with night driving due to the glare of oncoming headlights.

Opacification of the anterior subcapsular zone can also occur, resulting in *anterior subcapsular cataracts*. While much less common, these lens opacities can also be fairly debilitating if located on or near the visual axis.

Figure 1.11
A typical PSC, demonstrating the whitish plaquelike appearance on the visual axis.

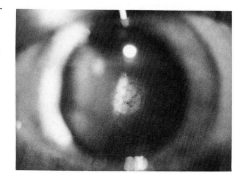

☐ Secondary (Complicated) Cataract

A cataract that results from another ocular disease process is termed a *secondary* or *complicated cataract*. These diseases include:

- Uveitis (Fuch's heterochromic iridocylitis, sarcoid, pars planitis)
- Hereditary retinal disorders (retinitis pigmentosa)
- Uncontrolled or end-stage glaucoma
- Rubeotic glaucoma
- Chronic retinal detachment
- Pathologic myopia

☐ Cataract Associated with Systemic Disease

Although not common, cataracts are sometimes an ocular manifestation of systemic disease:

1. Diabetes—Diabetics tend to develop typical age-related opacities at an earlier age than do nondiabetics. A true diabetic or *snowflake* cataract is rare (Figure 1.12).
2. Hypoparathyroidism (hypocalcemia)
3. Metabolic storage diseases
   a. Galactosemia
   b. Mannosidosis
   c. Fabry's disease
   d. Wilson's disease
   e. Lowe's syndrome
4. Myotonic dystrophy
5. Atopic dermatitis

☐ Drug-induced Cataracts

When used long-term, there are several drugs that can result in cataract formation:

Corticosteroids. Patients on long-term topical or systemic corticosteroids can develop PSC cataracts over time.

Phenothiazines. Patients with mental disorders on one of the phenothiazine derivatives (for example, Thorazine) may develop pigment deposition on the anterior lens capsule (Plate 4). These deposits rarely interfere with vision.

Figure 1.12
A true diabetic or *snowflake* cataract.

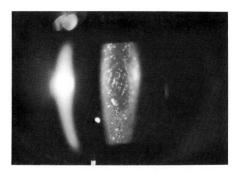

Miotics. Glaucoma patients on topical long-acting cholinesterase inhibitors (for example, phospholine iodide) can develop lens opacities. With the advent of newer glaucoma medications and laser procedures, these miotics are rarely used.

Mevacor (lovostatin) is a cholesterol-lowering drug used by many Americans. When it was first approved by the Food and Drug Administration (FDA), warnings went out to physicians on the drug's potential role in causing cataracts. Patients were encouraged to undergo a baseline slit lamp examination prior to starting the medication. To date, however, there is no convincing evidence to support these claims. A baseline examination is always a good idea, but patients should be reassured that the medication will not cause cataracts.

□ Traumatic Cataracts

The crystalline lens can become opacified or displaced as a result of trauma. These cataracts are most often unilateral and may be related specifically to:

Blunt trauma. A blunt injury to the eye can result in a *rosette-shaped cataract* that may progress further with time. With a more forceful injury, a denser opacity can result with or without subluxation (Figure 1.13).

Figure 1.13
A dense cortical cataract with subluxation inferiorly—secondary to blunt trauma to the eye with a fist. Note the iridodialysis superiorly.

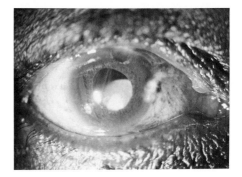

Penetrating injury. Direct injury to the lens itself due to a penetrating foreign body will usually result in the rapid formation of a cataract.

Radiation. Radiation to an eye, for example, following pterygium resection, can result in lens opacification.

Electric shock. Cataract following electric shock has been reported but is extremely rare.

___ ■_____

EPIDEMIOLOGY

Limited information is available on the frequency, distribution by age, and type of lens opacities that exist in the United States. This is in part due to differences in populations studied as well as to the lack of a standard clinical definition or a grading system for cataracts. Regardless, there are certain assumptions that can be made based on clinical experience and supported by recent literature:

- The older the patient, the greater the incidence of cataracts.
- NS is the most common age-related opacity followed by cortical changes. The least common opacity is PSC, although it is seen frequently in surgical practices due to its debilitating effect on acuity. Many patients will present with a combination of the three age-related changes.

Although it is difficult to determine the number of patients who develop age-related cataracts each year, information on the number of cataract surgeries performed is more easily obtained. Cataract surgery is the most frequently performed operation in the United States. (In 1991, it is estimated that between 1.4 and 1.5 million cataract procedures were performed.*) This number will most likely continue to increase in the future.

_____

*Health Products Research, Inc., Lewis Coopersmith, personal communication.

2

The Preoperative Evaluation

☐

Evaluating a patient with vision loss due to cataracts is similar to evaluating a patient with any ocular condition, with a few variations and additions.

A thorough and consistent examination should be performed on all patients regardless of the reason for the visit. Once a sense of the problem is determined, disease-specific tests can be added to the standard examination based on the history, the clinical findings, and the examiner's intuition and experience.

Care should be taken to avoid formulating a final decision before completing the examination, as clinicians sometimes tend to make the findings fit a predetermined diagnosis. By keeping an open mind and being watchful for multiple problems in a given patient, very little should go undetected.

A flow chart of a complete exam is shown in Figure 2.1. Those parts of the examination that are important in the preoperative cataract evaluation will be discussed in detail.

■ CASE HISTORY

The case history of a cataract patient is the foundation on which an appropriate assessment and treatment plan is built. The case history can be divided into:

Ocular history. Past and present

Medical history. Including medications

Family history. Ocular and medical

☐ Present Ocular History

A good ocular history, regardless of the particular problem, should be complete, concise, and chronological. As best possible, obtain the facts regarding the patient's

CASE HISTORY

Gradual progressive VA loss, unilateral or bilateral
Functional history: problems driving, reading, sewing, and getting around with
emphasis on outdoor versus indoor illumination, glare

History of ocular disease, trauma, medical history, medications, family history
↓
ENTRANCE ACUITY

Distance and Near
(with Pinhole)
↓
RETINOSCOPY/REFRACTION
↓
GLARE TESTING
↓
CONFRONTATION
VISUAL FIELDS
↓
MOTILITY
↓
PUPILLARY TESTING
↓
BIOMICROSCOPY
(pre-dilation)

Lids, lashes, conjunctiva, cornea, angle estimation A/C, iris and initial (brief) glance at
crystalline lens
↓
TONOMETRY
↓
GONIOSCOPY
(when indicated)
↓
* * * * * *
D I L A T I O N
* * * * * *
↓
POTENTIAL ACUITY TESTING
↓
BIOMICROSCOPY
(postdilation)

Thorough evaluation of crystalline lens, including 1. Grading opacity 2. Grading Hruby/
90D lens view through opacity
↓
FUNDUS EXAM

Evaluation of disc, macula, vessels, and periphery
↓
IMPRESSION
↓
PATIENT CONSULTATION AND FINAL PLAN

Figure 2.1   Flow chart of a suggested cataract evaluation.

vision loss and level of functioning. If the patient is a poor historian, ask family members to fill in missing information and to share observations regarding patient mobility and behavior.

BE COMPLETE

Do not assume that patients will volunteer information relevant to the case. It is the responsibility of the clinician to question the patient and investigate the problem thoroughly.

BE CONCISE

Once the facts are known, translate them into language that will be clearly understood, as if one were dictating a note to another physician summarizing the patient's problem.

Example

- 76 year old white female
- No ocular problems until two years ago when patient began noting gradual, progressive acuity loss OD > OS.
- She is no longer able to read or sew and has difficulty outdoors on sunny days.

RECORD CHRONOLOGICALLY

This will help establish a meaningful record of the problem(s) for years to come. Document dates of visits, doctors' names, diagnoses, and recommended treatment plans in the order in which they occurred.

A typical cataract history usually includes symptoms of painless visual acuity loss in one or both eyes, with slow progression over several months or years. Surprising numbers of patients with cataracts are unaware that their acuity is reduced, perhaps because of the gradual nature of the loss. Others will present with a reported sudden loss of visual acuity (VA) in one eye, which in reality represents a slowly progressive cataract that the patient suddenly noticed after accidentally covering the other eye.

Truly sudden loss of vision is of course inconsistent with cataract unless it is traumatically induced. Symptoms of discomfort or pain are also unlikely to be caused by the cataract unless they are related to extreme glare or to a hypermature lens with anaphylactic response.

Questions pertaining to the individual's ability to function on a daily basis are important. The answers to these questions often determine the need for surgery. (If the patient does not respond to an open-ended question such as, "What kind of problems are you having with your vision?" then specific areas should be explored.)

Ask if the patient is having problems with:

- Work-related tasks
- Reading
- Sewing/knitting
- Near work
- Hobbies
- Driving—day or night
- Glare from oncoming headlights
- Color desaturation
- Bright sunny days
- Mobility around the home
- Mobility in unfamiliar areas

□ Past Ocular History

Other ocular diseases, trauma, or a past history of ocular surgery should be noted and considered as possible underlying causes of the cataract. These entities include:

- Chronic uveitis (pars planitis, Fuch's heterochromic iridocylitis, sarcoidosis)
- Diabetic retinopathy
- Glaucoma
- Longstanding retinal detachment
- Retinitis pigmentosa and other hereditary retinal disorders
- Blunt trauma
- Penetrating injuries
- Trabeculectomy, vitrectomy, or penetrating keratoplasty surgery

While evaluating a cataractous eye, it is also important to be aware of any preexisting strabismic or anisometropic amblyopia. Even in the presence of a densely opaque lens, a patient who reports that the acuity has always been poor in that eye may not be a good candidate for surgery if there is little or no potential for improvement.

□ Medical History

The medical history of each cataract patient should also be thoroughly explored. A patient's health can affect development of cataracts and can also determine whether the patient is able to undergo a surgical procedure. Some of the systemic diseases that can be associated with formation of cataracts are:

- Diabetes
- Metabolic disorders such as galactosemia or hypoparathyroidism
- Chromosomal abnormalities such as Down's syndrome
- Congenital rubella

☐ Medications

Careful questioning regarding chronic use of medications or exposure to toxic substances may explain the presence of cataracts. Drugs to be particularly alert to include corticosteroids, phenothiazines, and miotics.

☐ Family History

Before one leaves the case history to begin the examination, brief questioning regarding family medical and eye history should be carried out. Most all patients will tell you that someone in their family has had cataract surgery in the past. This is usually not significant, however, unless the cataracts developed at a young age.

OCULAR EXAMINATION

☐ Entrance Acuity

Every examination, both initial and follow-up, should begin with visual acuity testing using some form of the Snellen chart. Many practitioners use projector charts and mirrors if the room is less than 20 feet in length. Acuity should be tested monocularly at distance, using the patient's habitual prescription in dim illumination. Any patient with VA less than 20/20 should be retested using the pinhole to determine the potential for refractive correction.

With the lights on, the near acuity should then be tested. Many patients rely on reading for their vocation and also as an important hobby and way to keep in touch with the world. Because any drop in near acuity can be extremely debilitating, checking near VA and comparing it with distance VA can be very useful. Depending on the type of cataract, distance and near acuity will usually be affected accordingly:

Nuclear sclerosis (NS). Distance vision reduced compared with near VA

Posterior subcapsular cataract (PSC). Near VA reduced compared with distance VA

In addition to reduced VA, cataracts may also be responsible for complaints of *ghost images,* also known as *monocular diplopia.* On questioning, patients may describe a starburst pattern around lights at night. This symptom may first be reported during VA testing and should be noted accordingly. The ghosting will usually disappear with the pinhole. Other causes of monocular diplopia include early keratoconus, epithelial basement membrane dystrophy, and irregular astigmatism following cataract or corneal surgery.

A technique that can be used to distinguish corneal from lenticular diplopia is to place a diagnostic hard contact lens of the appropriate base curve on an anesthetized eye and do an over refraction. If the monocular ghosting resolves and the vision improves, the etiology is probably corneal. If it does not, the etiology is probably lenticular.

□ Retinoscopy/Refraction

The refraction is performed, again with room lights dim, and the best corrected acuity is obtained. An issue that often arises is just how hard to push a patient when testing VA. There are two schools of thought on this:

1. Encourage patients to read the lowest line they can, urging them to guess letter-by-letter if they begin to hesitate. For example, a patient is pushed several lines beyond the threshold where they can easily read, say to 20/30. Subsequent examination of the crystalline lens reveals an early NS cataract consistent with 20/30 vision. If acuity was recorded at 20/50 but the lens looked consistent with 20/30, there would be two lines of acuity loss to explain. If the fundus was normal, further testing or referral would become necessary.

2. Record acuity when the patient *first* begins to note difficulty. This may be a more accurate reflection of their functional acuity, which of course is the most important factor in considering surgery.

A good compromise may be to record both the functional level (where the patient first has difficulty) and the level to which the patient can be maximally pushed, and record both on the examination form.

□ Glare Testing

Since a dimly lit examination room and a high contrast acuity chart do not represent a natural environment, it is important to retest patients under conditions that they are more likely to encounter. Glare, defined as light scatter resulting in a degraded retinal image and often extreme discomfort, is particularly troublesome to many cataract patients. Reasons for performing glare testing on cataract patients include:

- Quantifying the effects of glare on visual performance
- Obtaining additional information with which to make a decision regarding cataract surgery

• Providing documentation to peer review organizations (PRO) and insurance companies that acuity falls below a certain level in order for them to cover the procedure.

There are many forms of glare testing ranging from simple and inexpensive to complex and costly. The most common procedures and instruments include room-lights-on acuity, autorefractor glare testing, brightness acuity testing, and tabletop glare testing.

ROOM-LIGHTS-ON ACUITY

The simplest of glare tests involves turning the room lights on after measuring the patient's best corrected acuity. This and all glare testing should be done prior to dilation. Snellen acuity will either remain the same or drop to a poorer level.

$$\text{cc VA } 20/60 \xrightarrow{\text{lights on}} \text{no change}$$

or

$$\text{cc VA } 20/60 \xrightarrow{\text{lights on}} 20/200$$

This room-lights-on technique is quick, easy, and gives the practitioner a better idea of the patient's functional acuity.

AUTOREFRACTOR GLARE TESTING

Some autorefractors incorporate a glare testing feature consisting of a low contrast Snellen chart with a glare source above and below. Acuity is taken initially, then retaken with the glare source on (Figure 2.2).

BRIGHTNESS ACUITY TESTING

The Brightness Acuity Tester (BAT) by Mentor is a hand-held instrument consisting of a small white, Ganzfeld-like bowl that the patient looks through while viewing the Snellen chart (Figure 2.3). The bowl is illuminated at a low, medium, or high intensity setting, simulating indoor, partly sunny, and bright sunny lighting conditions respectively. The patient is then asked to re-read the chart, and any drop in acuity is recorded. This instrument is very useful for correlating patient symptoms to acuity loss in high-glare conditions.

TABLETOP GLARE TESTING

There are several commercially available tabletop testers that employ either central or peripheral glare sources. Among those available are the Titmus Miller-

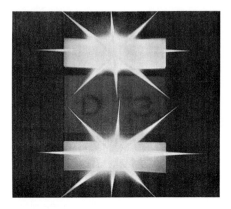

Figure 2.2
Some autorefractors have a built-in glare testing feature (photo courtesy of Humphrey Instruments, Inc.)

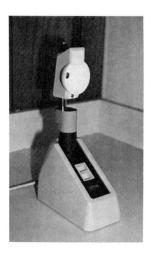

Figure 2.3
The Brightness Acuity Tester (BAT) by Mentor simulates various glare conditions, including partly sunny and bright sunny days.

Nadler Glare Tester, the Vistech MCT 8000 Multivision Contrast Tester, the Optec 1500 Glare Tester, and the Terry Vision Analyzer.

None of these testers is standardized, and all rely on subjective responses from patients. This does not make them any less valuable, however, in providing additional information to confirm patient symptoms and to justify surgical intervention that in the past might have been considered too early.

CONTRAST SENSITIVITY

There has been a great deal of emphasis placed on testing contrast sensitivity in patients with ocular disease, including cataracts. Testing is done with one of several charts commercially available, consisting of grating patterns of alternate light and dark stripes. Patients are asked to orient the stripes (vertical, horizontal, or oblique) as they become thinner (higher spatial frequency). A contrast sensitivity curve is

Figure 2.4
Recording confrontation fields.

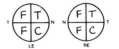

FTFC = full-to-finger counting

plotted based on test results, which provides information on the quality of vision at multiple contrast levels.

This test can be used to document the effects of early cataracts on visual performance over time. Despite the useful information it may provide, contrast sensitivity has not been widely used or accepted in evaluating the preoperative cataract patient.

□ Visual Fields

Screening confrontation fields should be part of every initial eye examination, including the preoperative cataract work-up (Figure 2.4). While cataracts may cause a generalized reduction in sensitivity over the entire field, they never cause quadrantic or hemianopic defects. Confrontation fields may be useful in detecting an early nasal step in low-tension glaucoma, or a homonymous hemianopsia in a stroke patient.

If confrontation fields are normal and there is no evidence of high intraocular pressure or pathologic cupping, formal automated perimetry is probably not necessary. If confrontation fields are abnormal or suspect, however, suprathreshold or threshold automated perimetry should be performed. Statistical analysis programs can aid the clinician in interpreting the results and distinguishing between generalized loss from media opacities and true field defects.

□ Motility

A careful cover test and thorough motility examination can reveal preexisting strabismus. A small angle esotropia, for example, might be the cause of amblyopia and reduced acuity in an eye that later develops a cataract. Conversely, a patient who develops a mature cataract can secondarily develop a sensory exotropia, although this is rare.

□ Pupillary Testing

Pupillary responses should be checked on all first-time patients and then once yearly. To avoid false positive results, an adequately bright light source should

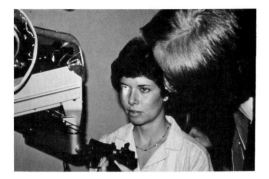

Figure 2.5
A binocular indirect
ophthalmoscope turned to
high is very useful in
pupillary testing.

			Direct	Consensual	
OD:	5.0mm	Blue	3+	3+	
					No afferent defect
					or
					− MG
OS:	5.0mm	Blue	3+	3+	

Table 2.1   An Example of Proper Pupillary Recording

be used. The binocular indirect ophthalmoscope (with the rheostat turned to high) is an excellent choice because of its strong concentrated beam of light and its accessibility in each examination room (Figure 2.5). Pupil size, iris color and direct/ consensual responses should be recorded in each eye rather than the standard but vague "PERRLA" notation. This should be followed by " ± APD", indicating afferent pupillary defect (also known as a *Marcus-Gunn pupil*) (Table 2.1). In the patient with a mature cataract, pupillary testing provides important information when a poor view of the fundus is obtained. A positive afferent defect signals the presence of optic nerve disease or extensive retinal damage.* In these cases, cataract surgery may not result in improved VA. Further testing such as B-Scan ultrasonography and electrophysiology is often useful in determining if surgery is indicated.

*Even a totally opaque crystalline lens *never* causes an afferent pupillary defect!

□ Slit Lamp Biomicroscopy

A complete slit lamp examination is an essential part of any cataract evaluation. It is important not only to look at the crystalline lens but also to detect any associated abnormalities.

Prior to dilation, a thorough assessment should be made of the lids, lashes, conjunctiva, cornea, anterior chamber, and iris. Chronic staph blepharitis should be treated preoperatively to lessen the risk of postoperative infection. Conjunctivitis or episcleritis should also be treated prior to the surgical referral. The cornea should be clear and the anterior chamber deep and quiet. Keratic precipitates (KPs) on the endothelium and anterior chamber cell and flare indicate uveitis that, if it is chronic, could be an underlying cause of cataract. Posterior uveitis caused by sarcoid or pars planitis is typically bilateral. Fuch's heterochromic iridocyclitis is a unilateral condition characterized by small stellate KPs located over the entire endothelium (Plate 5). The iris in the involved eye will often be lighter in color (Plate 6). This disorder commonly leads to development of cataracts and glaucoma.

In the case of an intumescent lens, the anterior chamber may be shallow and the angle approach narrow. Gonioscopy is extremely important as an adjunct to the slit lamp examination in these cases, in order to rule out chronic angle closure glaucoma. A shallow anterior chamber in conjunction with a symptomatic cataract may accelerate the need to perform surgery.

Following dilation, a thorough evaluation of the crystalline lens should be performed. Direct illumination as well as retroillumination should be utilized in carefully observing the type, location, and degree of lenticular opacification.

Various systems can be used to grade a lens opacity. The conventional 0 to 4 + scale is commonly employed. Zero denotes no opacity and 4 + indicates a totally mature cataract. For example, a moderate nuclear cataract might be graded as "2 + NS." While this scale serves as a gross method of quantifying the density of a given cataract, it should be used with the understanding that there will probably be significant interobserver variability.

Perhaps a more useful technique is to grade one's view of the fundus *through* the cataract rather than grading the cataract itself. For example, a patient with moderate 2 + NS has a best corrected acuity of 20/50. Using the Hruby or 90D fundus lens and biomicroscope, a somewhat blurred view of the retina and optic nerve is noted although most structures are still visible. This reduction in view could be considered moderate or 20/50 and consistent with the patient's VA. If, on the other hand, the patient's best corrected VA is 20/200, but the clinician's view through the same moderate NS is 20/50, look for other reasons for the acuity loss aside from the cataract. The patient may have a macular hole or other retinal abnormality that is responsible for the difference in acuity between 20/50 and 20/200.

The importance of assessing the role a cataract plays in vision loss cannot be overstated. Too often clinicians note VA loss, then note a cataract, and conclude

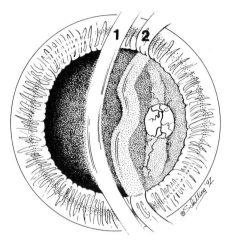

Figure 2.6
Using the biomicroscope and a fundus lens, the vertical slit beam (1) will look bowed *away from* the observer when it is directed through a milky NS cataract onto the retina (2). (Illustration by Stephanie Schilling)

that the VA loss is due to the cataract. It is the responsibility of every clinician to look beyond the lens to be sure the rest of the eye is healthy. Suspicion should be raised when the acuity, degree of opacification, and view of the fundus through the lens are inconsistent.

One of the few cases where the view of the fundus may be deceptively clear compared to the VA is with a variant of NS called *milky NS* (see Plate 2). Milky NS, with its characteristic lens-within-a-lens appearance, will allow a relatively clear view of fundus details despite its significant interference with vision. Confirmation that the cataract is the sole cause of the vision loss comes from the appearance of the slit lamp beam on the fundus. Using the Hruby, or 90 diopter, lens, the vertical beam will appear *bowed away from* the observer no matter where it is directed on the retina (Figure 2.6). This bowing of the beam indicates that the cataract, although it may not look significant, is probably responsible for the patient's reduced acuity. Milky NS will often cause a significant refractive shift as well. Three or four diopters of induced myopia is not unusual in early milky NS, and there have been changes as high as 10 diopters noted over a relatively short period of time.

The identification of subtle lens opacities, such as milky NS, can save the patient from an expensive and time-consuming search for unexplained VA loss. The following is an actual case that nicely illustrates this point:

A 52-year-old white female presented with a seven-month history of gradual painless vision loss in the right eye. After first noting the reduced vision, she saw an eye doctor who recorded best corrected visual acuity of 20/25 OD and 20/20 OS without any obvious explanation. The patient returned for several more office visits at which time visual fields and fluorescein angiography were performed. Because all test results were negative, the patient was referred to a local neurologist for evaluation. A magnetic resonance imaging (MRI) scan was ordered and was normal. The cause of the VA loss remained in question. The patient was monitored for several more months, became frustrated, and was referred to the author for another opinion.

Examination revealed best corrected acuity of 20/30 −2 OD and 20/20 OS. Refraction was OD: −0.50 = −0.50 × 180; OS: +1.00 = −0.50 × 180. Confrontation fields, motility, and pupils were entirely normal. Biomicroscopy revealed early milky NS OD. The view of the fundus with the Hruby lens was a clear 20/20, but the center of the slit beam was bowed posteriorly wherever it was directed on the retina. The fundus itself was unremarkable.

The point to be made from this case report is that early milky NS can be difficult to detect, especially during a cursory slit lamp exam. Keen observational skills are important as well as careful evaluation of the structures of one eye compared to the other. Additional clues in this case were the early myopic shift of the right eye and the distortion of the slit beam on the retina.

□ Tonometry

Intraocular pressure should be measured on all patients, regardless of age or reason for seeking care. If a patient has elevated intraocular pressure *and* a cataract, a number of possible etiologies exist:

Chronic open-angle glaucoma. In the absence of other findings, this is the most likely diagnosis. The cataracts are most likely unrelated to the glaucoma although both are aging changes. Any patient with longstanding open angle glaucoma, however, runs the risk of accelerated cataract formation.

Chronic angle-closure glaucoma. An intumescent lens can cause slow closure of an angle over time without any of the symptoms of acute angle closure. A laser peripheral iridotomy may be indicated followed by cataract extraction.

Acute angle-closure glaucoma. Although not usually associated with cataracts, an acute angle-closure attack can cause necrosis of lenticular tissue, resulting in white flecklike anterior subcapsular opacities. This condition is known as *glaukomflecken* (Figure 2.7).

Phacolytic glaucoma. A hypermature cataract may leak lens protein, which results in a chronic inflammatory response. This can lead to secondary glaucoma, necessitating immediate removal of the cataract.

Angle-recession glaucoma. Blunt trauma to the eye can cause damage to the trabecular meshwork as well as a cataract, resulting in glaucoma. The onset of the glaucoma may be delayed months to years after the injury. Whenever a unilateral cataract is seen in conjunction with high pressure, the patient should be questioned about previous blunt trauma or penetrating injuries.

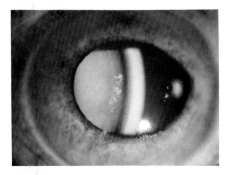

Figure 2.7
An acute angle-closure attack can cause necrosis of anterior capsular tissue known as glaukomflecken.

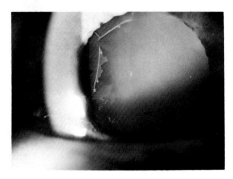

Figure 2.8
Pseudoexfoliation of the lens capsule.

Pseudoexfoliative glaucoma. Pseudoexfoliation of the lens capsule is character-ized by grayish-white deposits on the anterior lens capsule (Figure 2.8). Al-though the origin of these deposits is poorly understood, there is a significant association with glaucoma. If a cataract should develop as well, extreme care must be taken during surgery because the zonules are weaker and the posterior capsule is thinner. As a result, the risk of lens subluxation, IOL (intraocular lens) decentration, and vitreous loss are higher than they are in the average cataract patient.

Regardless of etiology, it is important to control the intraocular pressure *prior* to cataract surgery. None of the conditions mentioned in this section are necessarily contraindications to surgery.

☐ Potential Acuity Testing

Potential acuity testing can provide valuable information in the cataract patient when:

- There is coexisting retinal disease.
- The cataract is advanced enough to prevent a clear fundus view.
- Prognostic information on postoperative acuity is needed.

Figure 2.9
The Potential Acuity Meter (PAM) is mounted on a slit lamp, and its miniaturized Snellen chart is projected into the patient's eye.

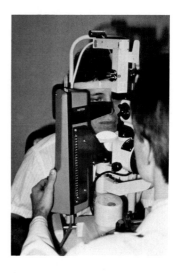

There are several instruments available that can aid in predicting postoperative acuity. These instruments vary in cost, accuracy, and ease of use. The results are subjective and should be taken in the context of the other examination findings. The instruments most commonly used are:

- Guyton-Minkowski Potential Acuity Meter
- Laser interferometer
- Bluefield Entoptoscope
- Super Pinhole™
- Maddox rod

POTENTIAL ACUITY METER

The Guyton-Minkowski Potential Acuity Meter (PAM) (Mentor, Inc.) is a portable instrument that mounts on most slit lamps (Figure 2.9). It predicts postoperative acuity in cataract patients by projecting a miniaturized Snellen acuity chart into the eye. The acuity achieved on this test is the acuity predicted following removal of the cataract. The instrument consists of an off/on switch, viewing window, and sphere power-control knob. To use it:

- Be sure the patient is dilated for best results.
- Align the patient in the slit lamp with the room lights off.
- Enter the patient's spherical equivalent prescription (Rx) into the instrument using the sphere power control.
- Looking around the slit lamp (the optics of the slit lamp are not used), aim the PAM beam into the patient's pupil. Focus in or out with the joystick until the patient reports seeing the Snellen chart.
- Ask the patient to read the lowest line possible. Because even the slightest head movement can obscure the target, the instrument should be adjusted

continuously during the examination to be sure the beam is being projected through an opening in the cataractous lens.

A poor response (PAM acuity *worse than* best corrected distance acuity) does not necessarily indicate that postoperative acuity will be poor. In the case of dense cataracts, the PAM beam may not penetrate through to the retina. In addition, some patients simply do not respond well to the test. When the PAM response is poor, however, extreme caution should be used before recommending surgery. Fundus findings, the status of the fellow eye, and clinical intuition will all enter into the final decision.

In patients whose PAM acuity is several lines *better than* their distance acuity, experience indicates that their postoperative acuity will usually improve to at least this level or often better.

Because it uses a Snellen chart, the PAM is easier for patients to respond to than are laser interferometers. It provides useful information in a majority of cases. It is relatively expensive, however, and is no longer reimbursable by Medicare and third-party carriers in many states.

LASER INTERFEROMETER

Laser interferometry uses two coherent light beams that project through the cataract onto the retina, producing a striped grid pattern that can be oriented vertically, horizontally, or obliquely. The finest grating pattern (least separation between lines) that the patient can correctly appreciate is converted to a Snellen equivalent and recorded as the potential acuity. Clinical interferometers, available in hand-held or slit lamp-mounted versions, can be more difficult for patients to respond to compared to reading the acuity chart in the PAM.

BLUEFIELD ENTOPTOSCOPE

The Bluefield Entoptoscope (Medical Instrument Research Associates, Inc.) takes advantage of the white corpuscle phenomenon to determine macular integrity and predict postoperative acuity. The instrument consists of a small portable box with a viewing port (Figure 2.10). The patient looks into the port and views cross hairs centered in a blue background. There is an off/on switch, a focusing knob, and light intensity controls. The test is performed by:

- Turning on the instrument and initially setting it on low or medium, depending on the density of the cataract. For extremely advanced opacities, the high setting is used.
- Focusing the cross hairs for each patient using the focusing knob.
- Asking the patients to describe what they see. They should respond by noting a blue background within which they see many moving *bugs, dots,* or *white specks.*
- Increasing the background intensity if they do not see the moving flecks, and giving the patient further prompting and instruction.

Figure 2.10
The Bluefield Entoptoscope is used to determine macular integrity before cataract surgery.

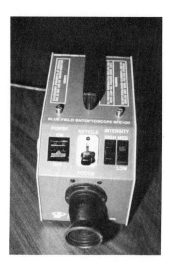

If they observe the phenomenon, there is a high probability that the patient will see 20/40 or better after surgery. In certain patients, however, such as those with a macular hole, the entoptic response may still be positive. This *false positive* result may mislead the clinician, emphasizing the importance of a thorough fundus evaluation.

If the patient *does not* observe the phenomenon, one of three possibilities exist:

1. The patient may not understand the test. Asking leading questions such as, "Do you see any moving dots?" may help prompt the response.

2. Some patients with the brunescent form of NS may not see the blue background. The brunescent lens can interfere with the transmission of blue light onto the retina, resulting in a *false negative* response.

3. The patient may have macular disease that prevents appreciation of the entoptic response.

SUPER PINHOLE

A less expensive device that seems to be gaining popularity is known as the *Super Pinhole*™. The instrument consists of a small box housing a transilluminated acuity chart, approximately 1000 times brighter than the standard Snellen chart (Figure 2.11). The patient, wearing pinhole spectacles, is asked to read the lowest line of the chart at a distance of 5 feet. After each eye is tested, the acuity is recorded. This acuity is then used to predict postoperative vision. The test is easy to perform and seems to be fairly accurate.

MADDOX ROD

Maddox rod orientation is a simple yet often effective way to grossly assess macular integrity. Place the maddox rod over the cataractous eye, present a bright light

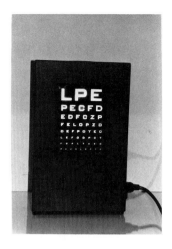

Figure 2.11
The Super Pinhole® device consists of a very
brightly lit acuity chart used with pinhole
glasses (photo courtesy of Robert B. Pinkert,
O.D.).

source, and ask the patient to identify the orientation of the red line. If they are
able to orient the line consistently and do not note gaps in the line, the macula
is probably fairly healthy.

The method chosen to test macular integrity and predict postoperative VA will
depend on the number of cataract patients seen, ease of use, and cost of instrumentation. The important factor to keep in mind is that none of these tests is
infallible, and all will produce false-positive and false-negative results. The information they provide must be taken in the context of the complete examination.

□ Fundus Examination

It is the responsibility of every primary care doctor of optometry to know what
is behind the lens before sending a patient for a surgical consult. This can only
be done with a careful, methodical dilated-fundus examination on every patient.
The fact that a patient has a cataract does not preclude that same patient from
also having a macular scar or glaucomatous cupping of the nerve head. Only by
being curious, suspicious, and observant will the clinician detect such abnormalities through the cataractous lens.

If retinal or optic nerve disease is detected, cataract surgery is not necessarily
contraindicated. The challenge for the doctor of optometry is to decide as accurately as possible what role the fundus anomaly is playing in the vision loss and
whether removing the cataract will leave the patient with a noticeable and useful
improvement in acuity. This decision in part will be made from experience and
in part will be based on results obtained from the testing described above.

3

The Surgical Decision

☐

Once the examination is completed and a diagnosis of cataract is made, the clinician must determine whether surgery will result in an improvement of vision (Figure 3.1). If the acuity loss is related to both the cataract *and* other ocular disease, it is important to assess the view of the fundus through the opacity and the results of potential acuity testing. Surgery should be recommended if some useful vision can be restored and if the patient's expectations are realistic.

If the acuity loss is related primarily to the cataract, the patient's lifestyle, visual demands, general health, and mental status should be considered. When the patient is no longer able to function optimally and must limit one or more activities, surgery can be recommended. If the patient seems to be getting along adequately, surgery should probably be deferred. By making the decision *with* the patient and not *for* the patient, the chance of a successful outcome is much higher.

These case histories illustrate that it is just as important to consider the individual's needs as it is their visual acuity (VA) and the appearance of the cataract.

Case Report 1

A 48-year-old male jeweler presented with a history of gradual VA loss in both eyes for six months. He finally sought help because he was unable to examine diamonds and other jewels, even with a ten-power loupe.

Examination revealed best corrected acuity of 20/25 OD and OS, dropping to 20/40 with room lights on. Near acuity was J7. Dilated slit lamp exam showed evidence of bilateral posterior subcapsular opacities, directly centered on the visual axis.

Despite his minimal VA loss, his livelihood was in jeopardy and surgery was recommended.

Case Report 2

A 92-year-old female presented for examination, stating her vision had become cloudy over the past year. She was in good health and did her own cooking and handiwork. She did not have much interest in reading but still enjoyed television.

Examination revealed best acuity of 20/60 OD and 20/50 OS. Near acuity was J5. Biomicroscopy revealed moderate nuclear sclerosis (NS) in both eyes. Fundus examination showed early drusen and atrophic age related macular changes.

Despite her moderate VA loss, she was functioning quite well. Surgery was deferred on this basis, with six-month follow-up visits recommended.

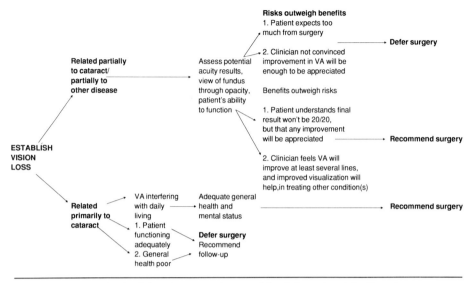

Figure 3.1   This decision tree can be used to determine whether to recommend cataract surgery.

Mental status is another consideration since some elderly patients are unable to explain their symptoms. Observations by relatives or friends may be helpful, especially regarding mobility and functioning. If the patient seems disoriented or confused, this is not necessarily a contraindication for surgery. There is a chance that the disorientation might be caused in part by the reduced vision and that surgery could make a difference. If there are doubts about the benefits of surgery, it is better to err on the side of caution and schedule a reevaluation.

In the case of cataract patients with co-existing ocular disease, careful evaluation and patient counseling are extremely important. Certain conditions that were once considered contraindications to cataract/implant surgery include:

- Diabetic retinopathy
- Open-angle glaucoma
- Chronic uveitis
- Retinal detachment
- A blind fellow eye

These disorders are no longer a reason to defer surgery, assuming that vision will improve somewhat. Successful surgery has been performed on many monocular patients and on patients with a variety of posterior segment diseases. In the case of diabetic retinopathy or advanced open-angle glaucoma, it is essential to explain clearly to the patient and family that the final visual result may not be 20/20. If the clinician feels that the patient will enjoy enough improvement in VA to make a difference in lifestyle, however, it may be worthwhile.

Another reason to recommend surgery in these cases is to allow better visualization of the fundus. This is critical in open-angle glaucoma in order to accurately evaluate the visual field and optic nerve head. A clear fundus view is also important in diabetes to closely monitor retinopathy and perform focal or panretinal laser photocoagulation if it is needed.

Uveitis is no longer an absolute contraindication to cataract surgery, although extreme caution must be used in deciding on the use of an implant. Active disease can complicate the postoperative result by clouding the implant with inflammatory debris. Preexisting cystoid macular edema may also be present, limiting the potential for sight.

A retinal detachment, once it is surgically repaired, is not a contraindication for cataract surgery. If peripheral retinal tears, holes, or lattice degeneration are present, these may need to be treated before surgery is scheduled.

INSURANCE APPROVAL

Familiarity with the VA and second opinion criteria of the major insurance carriers is helpful before making a surgical decision. Medicare and private companies are looking carefully at unnecessary surgery by scrutinizing preoperative acuity and test results. For a short period of time, Medicare patients had to be *precertified* for coverage through a state peer review organization (PRO). If the acuity was 20/50 or better, for example, the local Medicare intermediary would deny payment. Precertification was discontinued in 1991, but the state PROs remained intact and can review charts retrospectively at any time.

For patients under 65 with private insurance, the company may require a second opinion if the VA is better than a pretermined level. Unfortunately as of this writing, doctors of optometry are usually not recognized as second-opinion providers. This means that the surgeon of choice may have to send the patient to another surgeon for a second opinion. This results in increased costs and time spent by the patient and a second opinion that may conflict with the first.

EXPLAINING CATARACTS

No matter whether surgery is necessary, cataract patients should be given a careful explanation of the disorder. While the doctor of optometry knows that cataracts are benign and treatable, patients may have preconceived fears and misconceptions that should be addressed. Keep these thoughts in mind as patients are counseled.

Assess each patient's preexisting perception of what a cataract is, and tailor your explanation accordingly.

Some patients still think a cataract is a growth or film over the eye that must become ripe before it can be removed. Other patients have a much clearer understanding of the condition and are more interested in discussing specifics of treatment. A careful explanation by the doctor, along with diagrams and videotapes, will help educate the patient as to what a cataract is and how best to manage it. Describe it as a clouding of the normally clear human lens, similar to a dense smudge on an eyeglass lens. This cloudy lens must eventually be removed in order for sight to be restored.

Be sensitive and responsive to patient fears.

The first thing many patients think of when they experience reduced acuity is that it will lead to total blindness. The doctor's role is to provide reassurance that this is not the case and that vision loss from cataracts is reversible. If patients are not yet ready for surgery, they can be assured that delaying the procedure will not reduce the chances of success in the future.

Cataract patients, and for that matter any patients with ocular disease, may feel that using their eyes to read or watch TV will lead to further deterioration of the condition. It is important to educate them in this regard and encourage them to use their eyes as much as they need or want to.

___■_____

EXPLAINING SURGERY

Once a decision to proceed with surgery is reached, it is helpful and reassuring to explain to patients what is going to take place. They may have misconceptions regarding the cataract surgery itself, often from listening to family or friends. Even if they don't verbalize their concerns, it is helpful to raise these issues in order to allay their fears. A few of the most commonly asked questions include:

Will my cataract be removed with a laser?

This misconception probably has its origin in the early days of the YAG laser when some surgeons marketed its use in the treatment of posterior capsular opacification. Perhaps intentionally, vague advertising and patient word-of-mouth perpetuated the myth that cataract surgery is done with a laser.

If I'm awake during surgery, won't I feel the needles and experience pain?

Fear of pain is often what keeps people away from doctors' offices. Cataract patients are no different. People have been known to put off surgery for years, especially if they have heard horror stories from other patients about the long needles and painful injections. They can be reassured that a relaxing medication will be used prior to surgery to minimize any discomfort from the local injection.

In some situations, it may be comforting for the patient to talk to a past patient who has been through the same procedure. Keeping a list of past surgical patients who are willing to talk to prospective patients can be very helpful.

How long will I be out of work? What will I be restricted from doing, and for how long?

Patients still remember the stories from their parents or grandparents about the two-week hospital stays and sandbags on the head after cataract surgery. Although less and less common, there is an occasional fear that the procedure will disrupt the patient's routine for a significant period of time. Fortunately, they can be reassured that there will be minimal lost time from work and virtually no restrictions after surgery (see Chapter 5).

■

RECOMMENDING SECONDARY IMPLANTS

Until the mid to late 1970s, intraocular lenses were not commonly implanted at the time of cataract surgery. As a result, there are still some patients seen who are *aphakic*, wearing either a contact lens or aphakic spectacles. A secondary implant is often beneficial in eliminating one or more of these problems:

- Aphakic spectacle lens distortion
- Contact lens intolerance
- Inability to insert/remove/clean contact lenses
- Corneal hypoxia/pannus from contact lenses
- Desire not to deal with contact lenses

Secondary implants can be inserted successfully to provide improved quality of vision, lifestyle, and convenience for many patients. The type of intraocular lens (IOL) used depends on the type of surgery performed (see Chapter 4).

■

CHOOSING THE SURGEON

Doctors of optometry are in a unique position to make objective decisions that are in the best interests of their patients. Before sending a patient for cataract surgery, consider:

- Who is the most skilled surgeon available to perform the procedure?
- Does the surgeon do a fairly high volume of cases or just several per month?

In the best interest of your patient, a surgeon should be selected who is performing state-of-the-art procedures in a timely, efficient manner, with predictable and consistent results.

A few basic guidelines the practitioner can use to determine whether surgical results are predictable and consistent are:

Recovery of visual acuity within a reasonable time period. VA should be in the 20/25 to 20/200 range one day postoperatively and should improve steadily with each subsequent visit. Patients consistently presenting at the one or four week visits with VA less than 20/200 signal potential problems with the surgical technique. The type of procedure performed will determine the rate of visual recovery. Patients undergoing conventional planned extracapsular surgery will probably take longer to heal than will phacoemulsification patients who have had a scleral incision, and their vision, therefore, may not recover as quickly.

Final induced astigmatism under one diopter. With the advent of new surgical techniques and refinement of scleral incisions (see Chapter 4), induced post-operative astigmatism should be minimal. Larger limbal incisions are still used, however, and with them the increased likelihood of induced astigmatism. This should resolve on its own or by cutting sutures, but if it does not, your patients may not be receiving optimal care.

Minor complications seen only occasionally. Every surgeon will have the occasional patient with corneal edema, elevated intraocular pressure (IOP), microhyphema, or pain. If the doctor of optometry sees these or any other minor complications on a regular basis, however, questions must be raised about the quality of surgery.

Major complications seen only rarely. Intraoperative and postoperative complications such as vitreous loss, expulsive hemorrhage, endophthalmitis, pupillary distortion, or bullous keratopathy are rare. If these problems occur frequently, another surgeon should be selected.

Is there is a correlation between predictable, consistent results and the volume of surgery performed? It stands to reason that high volume surgeons doing 20 to

40 procedures per week have more experience and a higher skill level than do surgeons handling one to five cases per week. The high-volume surgeons tend to work more quickly and efficiently, usually in an outpatient surgery setting.

Questions that should also be asked include:

- Is the surgeon's philosophy on selecting surgical candidates consistent with my own?
- Is the surgeon ethical in every respect?

Predictable and consistent surgical results are not the only factors to consider. With more surgeons competing for the same surgical volume, unnecessary surgery is unfortunately being performed. Patients who are told they *must* have surgery or who are being scheduled without any obvious visual complaints may not be in the best of hands. Be sure the surgeon is honest and ethical in dealing with patients and co-managing doctors of optometry:

- Is the surgeon cooperative, communicative, and available to me and my patients?
- Is the surgeon willing to co-manage surgical patients and actively involve me in postoperative care?

These two issues go hand-in-hand. The referring doctor should expect detailed and timely communication from the surgeon regarding the patient's status. The surgeon, in turn, should be comfortable with the postoperative diagnostic and management skills of the optometrist. An initial meeting may be necessary to establish clinical protocols so that each professional knows what the other expects.

PRESURGICAL TESTING

Once the patient is referred for surgery, certain tests will be done in preparation for the procedure. Surgeons will probably repeat some of the basic tests for their records along with the ancillary tests necessary for surgery, which include:

Keratometry. These readings are needed as baseline preoperative information as well as for the intraocular lens (IOL) power calculation.

A-scan ultrasound. This instrument measures the axial length of the eye, the results of which are needed to determine the appropriate IOL power (Figure 3.2).

B-scan ultrasound. This test is needed if the cataract is so mature that a poor view or no view of the fundus is obtained. The B-scan can only rule out elevations

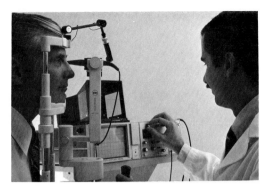

Figure 3.2
A-scan ultrasonography measures the axial length of the eye, used to determine the power of the IOL.

or depressions of the fundus such as retinal detachment, melanoma, or advanced glaucomatous cupping. It will typically *not* detect atrophic macular degeneration or macular edema.

Specular microscopy. This instrument evaluates the density and integrity of corneal endothelial cells, thus helping to predict how well the cornea will tolerate the trauma of intraocular surgery. Specular microscopy is particularly useful when phacoemulsification is planned and the patient has a history of corneal decompensation in the fellow eye, or the presence of guttata or other corneal dystrophy is noted. The equipment consists of an applanation device, a screen, and a video recorder (Figure 3.3) and is fairly costly. An inexpensive alternative is to estimate the endothelial cell count using specular reflection with a slit lamp. A special reticule can be inserted in the eyepiece of a bio-microscope to aid in counting the density of cells per square millimeter. Normal counts are usually over 2000 cells per square millimeter. Counts of 1000 to 2000 are considered borderline, depending on the shape and consistency of the cells.

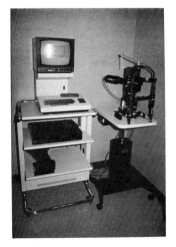

Figure 3.3
Specular microscope with video recorder.

Counts below 1000 are abnormally low. Low or borderline cell counts do not necessarily contraindicate surgery but allow the doctor to alert the patient to possible corneal complications in the future.

■ SURGICAL SCHEDULING

Most large surgical practices have designated staff who schedule surgery and counsel patients on all aspects of the procedure and on insurance coverage. Brochures, educational videotapes, and written instructions can be used (Figure 3.4). The co-managing doctor of optometry should be thoroughly familiar with the surgeon's preoperative protocol should the patient call with questions. The more knowledgeable and less anxious the patient is, the more pleasant the experience will be.

■ INFORMED CONSENT

Before surgery is performed, the patient is asked to sign an informed consent document (Figure 3.5). This form reviews pertinent facts related to surgery, including the purpose of the procedure and all possible risks related to the procedure. By signing the form, the patient gives the surgeon permission to perform the operation. Regulations regarding informed consent vary by state and medical community.

■ MEDICAL CLEARANCE

Anesthesiologists at most hospitals and surgical centers require a basic medical evaluation prior to surgery. The extent of the work-up varies considerably based on the standards of care in the community. It may be done in the surgeon's office by a physician's assistant or a nurse, by the patient's medical doctor, or in an outpatient surgical center or hospital by the anesthesia staff.

Some tests that may be ordered include:

- History and physical examination
- Complete blood count (CBC) and electrolytes

PAUL C. AJAMIAN, O.D., F.A.A.O.
Center Director

RALPH C. DiIORIO, M.D.
Medical Director

OMNI EYE SERVICES

OUTPATIENT SURGERY
Pre-Op Instructions

IMPORTANT INFORMATION FOR: _____

AM
You have been scheduled for outpatient surgery at _____PM on_____.

AM
Please report to our office **FIRST**, promptly at _____PM. The address is: 5505 Peachtree-Dunwoody Road, Atlanta, 3rd Floor, Suite 300.

Your first postoperative visit will be in our office the day after surgery. The time will be given to you on the day of surgery.

PRE-OP INSTRUCTIONS

1. An eye drop and an ointment will be prescribed. Please start using these in your _____ eye on _____

   _____, 3 days before surgery.

   DETAILED INSTRUCTIONS: Gentamicin (Genoptic) drops: Use in the _____ eye three (3) times a day three days before surgery. Polysporin Ointment: Use by applying to your eye lids (upper & lower) at bedtime, 3 days before surgery.

   NOTE: Save the **drops** as you will be using these after surgery as well.

2. Do not eat or drink anything after midnight the night before your surgery. Do not eat or drink anything the morning of your surgery.

3. You may take your regular oral medications with a sip of water.

4. If you are an insulin dependent diabetic **do not take the insulin on the day of surgery.**

5. Please make arrangements (unless you are coming on our van) to have a family member or friend with you. This person should be available to take you home. Since the waiting room is small, please try to limit the number of people you bring to one or two.

6. The pre-op physical exam, blood work and EKG may be done in our office prior to or on the day of surgery. If you did not or do not plan to have these tests done in our office, please bring all required test results with you on the day of surgery.

   THANK YOU FOR YOUR COOPERATION! CALL US IF YOU HAVE ANY QUESTIONS AT
   257-0814 or 1-800-822-4585 (Georgia WATS)

Instructions given by: _____ Date Sent: _____

_____

I understand and assume responsibility for following the above instructions.

SIGNED: _____ DATE: _____

Figure 3.4 Written instructions for the preoperative cataract patient.

INFORMED CONSENT FOR CATARACT AND/OR INTRAOCULAR LENS SURGERY

INTRODUCTION - THIS INFORMATION IS GIVEN TO YOU SO YOU CAN MAKE AN INFORMED DECISION ABOUT HAVING EYE SURGERY. TAKE AS MUCH TIME AS YOU WISH TO MAKE YOUR DECISION ABOUT SIGNING THIS CONSENT. YOU HAVE THE RIGHT TO ASK QUESTIONS ABOUT ANY PROCEDURE BEFORE AGREEING TO HAVE AN OPERATION.

EXCEPT FOR UNUSUAL PROBLEMS, A CATARACT OPERATION IS INDICATED ONLY WHEN YOU FEEL YOU CANNOT FUNCTION ADEQUATELY DUE TO POOR SIGHT PRODUCED BY A CATARACT, WHICH IS A CLOUDY NATURAL LENS INSIDE THE EYE. THE NATURAL LENS WITHIN YOUR OWN EYE THAT HAS A SLIGHT CATARACT, ALTHOUGH NOT PERFECT, HAS SOME ADVANTAGES OVER ANY MAN-MADE LENS.

YOU AND YOUR DOCTOR ARE THE ONLY ONES WHO CAN DETERMINE IF OR WHEN YOU SHOULD HAVE A CATARACT OPERATION - BASED ON YOUR OWN VISUAL NEEDS AND MEDICAL CONSIDERATIONS.

ALTERNATIVE TREATMENTS - I understand I may decide not to have a cataract operation at all. However, should I decide to have an operation, I understand these are the three methods of restoring useful vision after the operation.

1. SPECTACLES (GLASSES) - Cataract spectacles required to correct your vision are usually thicker and heavier than conventional eyeglasses. Cataract spectacles increase the size of objects about 25% and clear vision is obtained through the central part of cataract spectacles which means you must learn to turn your head to see clearly on either side. Cataract spectacles usually **CANNOT** be used if a cataract is removed in **ONE EYE** and the other is normal, because they may cause double vision.

2. CONTACT LENS - A hard or soft contact lens increases the apparent size of an object about 8%. Handling of a contact lens is difficult for some individuals. Most lenses must be inserted and removed daily or weekly and not everyone can tolerate them. For near tasks, eyeglasses (not cataract spectacles) are usually required in addition to contact lens.

3. INTRAOCULAR LENS (IOL) - This is a small plastic artificial lens surgically placed inside the eye permanently. With the intraocular lens there is little apparent change in the size of objects seen. Conventional eyeglasses (not cataract spectacles) are usually required in addition to the intraocular lens.

CLINICAL INVESTIGATION - The United States Food and Drug Administration (FDA) requires an ongoing clinical investigation of intraocular lenses to establish facts about safety and efficacy. I understand the study involves a minimum one-year observation of the results of my surgery whether a lens is implanted or not. The purpose of this observation is to compare in a similar group of patients the differences, if any, in eyes with and without lens implantation and the differences, if any, between different styles of intraocular lenses. Information about the results of my surgery will be made available to the FDA. Confidentiality will be maintained. If for any reason I wish to decline participation in the study, I may do so without affecting my future care. It is estimated that ten million individuals have received intraocular lenses as patients in this study.

CONSENT FOR OPERATION - In giving my permission for a cataract extraction and/or for the possible implantation of an intraocular lens in my eye, I declare I understand the following information:

With Cataract Surgery I Have Approximately:

94-95% Chance of Better Vision — 1 out of 1000 Chance of Loss of Sight — 1% Chance of Useless Vision — 1% Chance of Retinal Detachment — 0.3% Chance of Infection — 5% Chance of Swelling of Retina — 10% Per Year Chance of Needing Yag Laser Treatment

If I decide to have an operation, I agree to have the type of operation listed below on my_____eye which I have indicated by my signature. Date_____.

(1) I wish to have a cataract operation with an intraocular lens._____
Patient's Signature

(2) I wish to have a cataract operation without an intraocular lens._____
Patient's Signature

(3) Since my cataract was previously removed and I have been informed by the doctor that my eye is medically acceptable for lens implantation, I wish to have an intraocular lens implanted._____
Patient's Signature

(4) I wish to have a lens implant removal, exchange or repositioning._____
Patient's Signature

NAME_____AGE_____

PLACE SIGNED_____

WITNESS' SIGNATURE _____ DOCTOR'S SIGNATURE _____
If you have any questions, please call our patient counselor at

Figure 3.5   Informed consent document for cataract surgery.

- Fasting blood sugar (for diabetics)
- Prothrombin time (for patients on anticoagulants)
- Electrocardiogram (EKG) (for patients with histories of heart disease)
- Chest X-ray (for patients with histories of emphysema or chronic obstructive pulmonary disease)

Any or all of these tests may be required, depending on the protocols established by the particular anesthesiologist and the surgical center.

ANESTHESIA ORDERS

The anesthesiologist usually sets policy regarding eating and drinking restrictions prior to surgery. Whether using local or general anesthesia, most anesthesiologists require the patient to be NPO (*nil per OS* [mouth]) after midnight before surgery; in other words, no solid food and no liquids allowed after midnight. The only exception is use of just enough water the morning of surgery to take regular systemic medications.

As a rule, patients about to undergo cataract surgery should continue taking all their systemic medications except:

Insulin and oral hypoglycemic agents. The use of injectable and oral hypoglycemic agents should be discontinued the night before surgery. Because patients will be fasting after midnight, the medications can cause severe *hypoglycemia* on the day of surgery. Special care is usually taken to schedule diabetic patients as early in the morning as possible so they can resume a normal eating schedule as soon as possible.

Blood thinners. Blood thinning agents such as Coumadin are usually discontinued three to five days prior to surgery to reduce the chances of uncontrolled bleeding during the procedure. Some surgeons also ask patients to avoid using aspirin prior to surgery.

PREOPERATIVE MEDICATION

Many surgeons believe in pretreating their surgical patients with topical antibiotic drops or ointment. The goal is to create a sterile environment that will prevent introduction of pathogenic bacteria into the eye at the time of surgery. A typical regimen includes use of a topical antibiotic drop three to four times a day for several days prior to surgery. For added safety, some surgeons also recommend a broad-spectrum antibiotic ointment along the lids at bedtime. Antibiotics commonly used include aminoglycosides (neomycin, gentamicin, or tobramycin), fluoroquinilones (Ciloxan or Chibroxin), and polysporin or erythromycin ointment. Some surgeons also pretreat the eye several hours before surgery with a topical nonsteroidal agent called Ocufen (flurbuprofen) that may inhibit miosis of the pupil during surgery.

THE SURGICAL FACILITY

While the choice of surgical facility has traditionally been viewed as beyond the control of the referring optometrist, it may be another factor in deciding which surgeon to use. There are four surgical settings available:

1. Hospital-inpatient facility
2. Hospital-outpatient facility
3. Freestanding outpatient surgical center
4. Surgery suite in doctor's office

In the early 1980s, the Health Care Financing Administration (HCFA) began requiring that all cataract patients covered by Medicare have their surgery performed on an outpatient basis. Most private insurance carriers adopted this requirement as well, virtually eliminating reimbursement for inpatient hospital stays except when it was medically necessary. As a result, cataract surgery shifted from a hospital inpatient procedure to an outpatient procedure in a short period of time. Another trend has been the shift from the hospital outpatient setting to the freestanding outpatient (ambulatory) surgical center setting. The advantages of this type of facility are:

Environment. A homelike atmosphere is provided, without the typical sterility of a hospital. Many patients associate hospitals with sickness and death, thus creating unnecessary anxiety. The center's staff is well trained to deal specifically with cataract patients and is able to respond to their needs and concerns.

Convenience. These centers are either in the same location as the surgeon's practice or nearby, allowing for easy access. Scheduling is often faster and more flexible because there is more direct communication between the practice and center. There is typically less red tape and more personalized attention when dealing with the staff of an outpatient surgery center as compared to a hospital.

Cost. The average facility fee for a freestanding surgical center is typically less than that for a hospital outpatient surgery center, and significantly less than for an inpatient hospital visit. The lower the facility fee, the less out-of-pocket expense to the patient no matter whether they have health insurance.

Some insurance carriers will only pay the facility fee if the surgery is done in a hospital outpatient center. Certain medical conditions such as recent heart surgery or renal dialysis may necessitate an inpatient hospital stay.

4

The Surgical Procedure

☐

In order to have a complete understanding of the pseudophakic eye and to provide the best pre- and postoperative care available, the doctor of optometry should be familiar with the latest surgical techniques. There are many variations of the basic cataract extraction, and it would be laborious to review all of them. The purpose of this chapter is to provide an overview of the entire surgical process, including cataract surgery as we know it today.

The reader is strongly encouraged to accompany several patients to surgery and to observe the entire process from beginning to end, including anesthesia, surgery, and recovery. The advantages of doing so include:

- Appreciation of what patients go through on surgery day
- Ability to counsel future cataract patients more knowledgeably
- Assessment of surgeon's technique, confidence level, management of intraoperative problems, and manner with patients
- Goodwill generated by being with the patients on surgery day, thus demonstrating commitment to every aspect of their care

■ ANESTHESIA

☐ Local Anesthesia

Local anesthesia is much more commonly used than general anesthesia is for cataract surgeries performed in the United States. There are many advantages:

- Conducive to an outpatient surgery setting
- Quick recovery period
- Reduced incidence of nausea and vomiting
- Reduced postoperative pain due to residual local anesthesia around the eye

Anesthesia in the outpatient setting is typically administered by such health care professionals as:

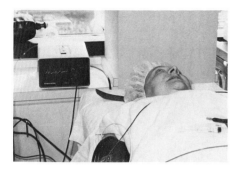

Figure 4.1
The patient is monitored during surgery using a pulse oximeter.

- An ophthalmic surgeon
- An anesthesiologist
- A certified registered nurse anesthetist (CRNA)
- A physician's assistant (PA)

Local anesthesia patients are monitored carefully before and during surgery just as general anesthesia patients are. Intraoperative monitoring is performed using a pulse oximeter (Figure 4.1), which monitors pulse rate and oxygen saturation in the blood, and an electrocardiogram (EKG). Anesthesiologists are usually available even if they are not actually administering the anesthesia.

There are several steps involved in the administration of local anesthesia, and as with the surgery itself, there are a number of possible variations. Each surgeon and anesthesiologist has a preference that can be learned by visiting their surgery center. One protocol commonly used is:

Mild sedation. An intravenous line is inserted and the patient is premedicated with a mild sedative, muscle relaxer and antianxiety agent such as Versed, Valium, Pentothal, Sublimaze, or Fentanyl. Some of these agents, like Versed, also cause short-term amnesia, so the patient does not remember the pain associated with the retrobulbar injection.

Orbicularis paralysis. The facial nerve is blocked to immobilize the orbicularis muscle of the eyelid and prevent squeezing during the surgery. This is accomplished with an injection of 2 percent lidocaine, given just under or in front of the ear (Figure 4.2).

Retrobulbar block. The goal of retrobulbar anesthesia is (a) to eliminate sensation to the conjunctiva, cornea, and uvea by blocking the ciliary nerves and (b) to immobilize the extraocular muscles by blocking the oculomotor (cranial nerve III), trochlear (cranial nerve IV), and abducens (cranial nerve VI) nerves. This is accomplished by depositing a bolus of anesthetic *behind* the globe within the muscle cone. An initial injection may be given to numb the lower lid area, which will reduce the sensation of the retrobulbar needle. Next a mixture of lidocaine (Xylocaine) and bupivicaine (Marcaine) is injected into the retrobulbar

Figure 4.2
A facial-nerve block is given to
immobilize the lids.

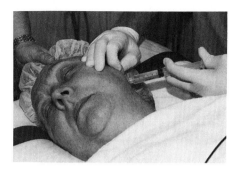

space by carefully directing the needle along the orbital floor under the globe
itself (Figure 4.3). The lidocaine and bupivicaine are mixed with hyaluronidase,
which promotes the spread of these drugs into the muscle cone and surrounding
orbital tissues. Lidocaine is a fast-onset but short-acting anesthetic, which is
why it is mixed with the longer-acting bupivicaine. The longer-acting agent
wears off slowly, keeping the patient free of pain during the immediate 24-hour
recovery period. Occasionally, however, the anesthesia wears off more rapidly,
and the patient may need an oral analgesic such as Tylenol with codeine.

□ Complications of Local Anesthesia

While the anesthesia just described is usually performed safely and routinely,
there are occasional complications that range from annoying nausea to devastating
vision loss. These complications include:

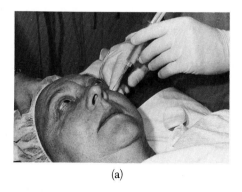

(a)

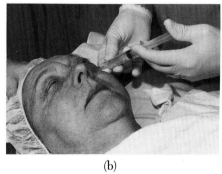

(b)

Figure 4.3 The retrobulbar injection is usually given at the inferior orbital
rim (a), and the needle is then directed under the eye along the
orbital floor (b).

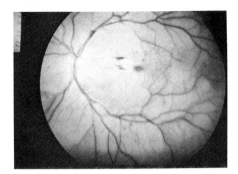

Figure 4.4
Central retinal artery occlusion as a result of retrobulbar injection into the optic nerve. The vision dropped to light perception only.

Retrobulbar hemorrhage. This fairly common complication occurs by some estimates in as many as one to two percent of patients undergoing retrobulbar injection. It is caused by the retrobulbar needle piercing one of the ciliary arteries or veins. Signs of a retrobulbar hemorrhage include progressive proptosis, conjunctival chemosis, subconjunctival hemorrhage, or elevated IOP (intraocular pressure). On recognition of such an orbital hemorrhage, surgery is usually postponed. The problem usually resolves quickly on its own.

Perforation of the globe. More common in highly myopic eyes, this rare complication can lead to retinal detachment and vitreous hemorrhage. The patient usually experiences severe pain.

Optic nerve damage. The retrobulbar needle can cause direct mechanical trauma to the optic nerve, resulting in ischemia and eventual optic atrophy. Vision loss can be devastating and is usually permanent.

Central retinal artery occlusion. Inadvertent injection of anesthetic into the nerve and central retinal artery can lead to a central retinal artery occlusion with immediate and permanent vision loss in the range of hand motion to light perception (Figure 4.4).

Central nervous system (CNS) toxicity. Local anesthetics injected into the orbit can diffuse into cerebrospinal fluid via the optic nerve. This is termed *central spread* and can result in symptoms of agitation, disorientation, nausea, vomiting, convulsions, and cardiac or respiratory arrest. Excessive doses of *any* local anesthetic can cause these and other complications.

☐ Alternatives to Retrobulbar Anesthesia

The complications associated with retrobulbar anesthesia, although rare, have led some surgeons to use an alternate method known as *periocular* or *peribulbar anesthesia.* This technique involves one or more injections around the globe, just past the equator (Figure 4.5). The technique is reportedly safer due to the fact that the needle remains further away from the globe, muscle cone, and optic

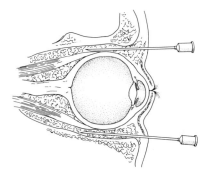

Figure 4.5   Peribulbar anesthesia with injection of anesthetic above and
below the globe just behind the equator. (Reprinted with
permission of the publisher from Davis DB, Mandel, MM
Peribular Anesthesia. *Regional Anesthesia for Intraocular
Surgery* 3, no. 1 [March 1990].)

nerve. Periocular injections are also less painful, and easier for some to perform.
The disadvantages of this relatively new procedure are the longer time it takes to
achieve adequate anesthesia and the higher volume of anesthetic needed. An
increasing number of surgeons are using this new form of local anesthesia. Due
to inexperience with this technique, however, the majority are still using retrobulbar anesthesia.

□ General Anesthesia

General anesthesia, although it is rarely used, is still a viable alternative for some
cataract patients such as children or people with Parkinson's disease who cannot
lie still during surgery. It is also useful for extremely nervous or anxious patients
who might otherwise not elect to undergo surgery. Many outpatient surgical
centers are equipped for general anesthesia as are all hospital outpatient centers.
Patients are still able to go home within a few hours after the surgery.

□ Final Preparations

After the retrobulbar or peribulbar block is administered, the patient is asked to
move the eye into all positions of gaze. Inability to do so indicates adequate
anesthesia. Before the patient is wheeled into the operating room from the preoperative area, final preparations are made:

   Reducing IOP. The eye must be softened prior to surgery to prevent vitreous
   loss and other complications. This can be done using:

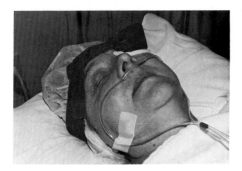

Figure 4.6
A mercury bag is placed on the eye for 20 to 30 minutes prior to surgery to lower the intraocular pressure. A nasal catheter will deliver oxygen to the patient once surgery begins.

Pressure on the globe. Pressure is applied to the eye either digitally or more commonly with a weighted device such as a mercury bag (Figure 4.6), a ball, or a Honan balloon. The device is typically kept on the eye for 20 to 30 minutes, and is the most effective and commonly used technique to lower IOP.

Medication. Oral or injectable agents can effectively lower IOP preoperatively although their use is limited. Medications include hyperosmotic agents such as glycerin or mannitol and carbonic anhydrase inhibitors such as acetazolamide (Diamox).

Anesthesia. Adequate retrobulbar anesthesia will prevent the patient from squeezing, which will keep the intraocular pressure low.

Oxygen supply. Since the patient's entire face will be covered with a drape during surgery, oxygen is supplied using a nasal catheter (see Figure 4.6). This provides reassurance to patients that they will be able to breathe adequately under the drape.

It is at this point that the patient is wheeled into the operating room. The skin surrounding the eye is disinfected using an iodine/soap solution (such as Betadine). The drape is put in place with only a small opening over the eye that is being operated on. The eyelids are retracted using a speculum (Figure 4.7). Some

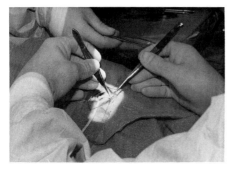

Figure 4.7
The patient's face is draped, leaving only the eye to be operated on exposed. A speculum holds the lids open while the surgeon prepares to suture the superior rectus muscle.

Figure 4.8
A bridle suture is placed through the superior rectus muscle anchored to the drape. This will keep the eye positioned downward, allowing for easier access into the anterior chamber.

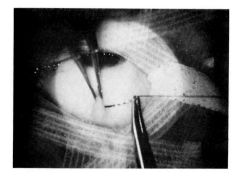

surgeons will then place a suture under the superior rectus muscle and anchor it onto the drape above the eye (Figure 4.8). The purpose of this *bridle suture* is to stabilize the eye and rotate it slightly downward for better access to the superior limbus. The surgeon, using an operating microscope, is now ready to begin the operation (Figure 4.9).

■ SURGICAL TECHNIQUES

□ Intracapsular Cataract Extraction (ICCE)

This technique is being reviewed primarily for historical purposes. While it is no longer commonly used in the United States, it is still widely practiced in Third World countries:

- A large limbal incision is made from 10 to 2 o'clock. This is often done by first making a partial thickness groove with a knife and then completing the

Figure 4.9
Using an operating microscope, the surgeon is ready to begin. (Courtesy of Ralph C. DiIorio, MD, and Atlanta Outpatient Surgery Center.)

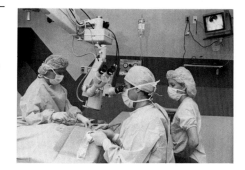

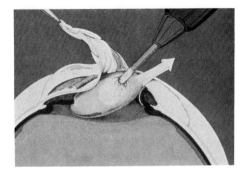

Figure 4.10
ICCE. (Courtesy of Allergan Medical Optics.)

opening with scissors. This opening will allow for removal of the entire crystalline lens.

• The zonules are dissolved by injecting an enzyme called alpha-chymotrypsin into the posterior chamber. This permits easier removal of the lens, especially in young patients.

• Using a disposable cryoprobe, the *entire* lens is removed from the eye (Figure 4.10).

• If an implant is to be used, it is placed in the anterior chamber.

• The incision is sutured closed.

□ Pars Plana Lensectomy

Removal of a cataract through the pars plana is usually performed by a retinal surgeon using vitrectomy instrumentation. Indications include congenital cataracts in children, traumatic cataracts with subluxation, or cataracts caused by longstanding uveitis with significant posterior synechiae.

□ Extracapsular Cataract Extraction (ECCE)

This surgical technique involves removal of the nucleus, either by physical expression or ultrasonic fragmentation. It has many advantages over intracapsular extraction, including:

• *Preservation of the posterior capsule,* which acts as a barrier preventing vitreous movement into the anterior chamber. This reduces the risk of complications such as retinal detachment, cystoid macular edema, and corneal decompensation from vitreous touch.

• *The ability to implant a posterior chamber intraocular lens,* the safest and most stable intraocular lens available.

Figure 4.11
ECCE. An anterior capsulotomy is performed by making small radial cuts in the anterior capsule. (Courtesy of Matthew J. Garston, O.D.)

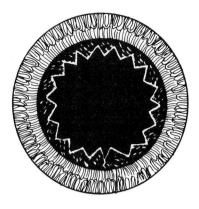

PLANNED EXTRACAPSULAR CATARACT EXTRACTION (ECCE)

The six basic steps involved with this technique are:

1. A bent needle inserted through a limbal opening is used to make a series of radial cuts in the anterior capsule. This anterior (or "can-opener") capsulotomy creates a 360° opening that will allow for removal of the nucleus (Figure 4.11).

2. A 10mm to 12mm incision is made at or slightly posterior to the limbus, using the technique described for intracapsular surgery.

3. The lens nucleus is expressed from the eye (Figure 4.12).

4. The cortex is now ready to be removed, using an irrigation-aspiration handpiece. This instrument infuses a balanced salt solution into the anterior chamber, keeping it well formed. The residual cortical material is then stripped and removed

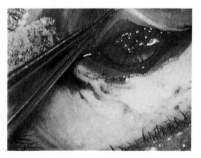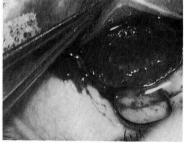

Figure 4.12   ECCE. The nucleus is expressed from the eye. (Courtesy of Ralph C. DiIorio, MD.)

from the eye (Figure 4.13). Extreme care must be taken to avoid rupturing the posterior capsule.

5. The posterior capsule itself must now be cleaned or *polished*. This is accomplished using a roughened instrument that removes any residual subcapsular opacities.

6. At this stage, the posterior chamber lens is inserted, and the wound is closed. (See the section titled "Insertion" later in this chapter.)

PHACOEMULSIFICATION

Phacoemulsification is a refined version of extracapsular surgery. The cataract is removed through a small incision by breaking up (emulsifying) the nucleus *inside* the eye, thereby eliminating the need for a large opening. Because this technique requires a high level of skill and experience, only a small percentage of surgeons have used it. A growing number of surgeons are becoming proficient, however, as the trend moves toward smaller incisions. Advantages of phacoemulsification over the conventional extracapsular technique include:

- Better control of the eye during surgery, allowing for rapid removal of instrumentation and wound closure in the event of an emergency
- More rapid healing because the wound is smaller
- Fewer patient restrictions after surgery and earlier resumption of professional and avocational activities
- More rapid recovery of vision with better uncorrected visual acuity due to less induced astigmatism
- Earlier stabilization of the spectacle prescription and thus fewer prescription changes
- Less likelihood of traumatic wound rupture postoperatively

Mastery of this technique is the basis for one-stitch and no-stitch surgery and for the implantation of foldable lenses as will be discussed later in this chapter.

Contraindications to performing phacoemulsification include:

A hard lens nucleus. The older the patient and the more brunescent the cataract, the more difficult it is to emulsify the nucleus ultrasonically. With the advent of viscoelastic substances to protect the cornea, this is less of an issue in the hands of a skilled phaco surgeon.

Corneal endothelial disease. With preexisting guttata or endothelial cell loss, phacoemulsification can further damage the endothelium resulting in decompensation of endothelial cells and resultant bullous keratopathy. The highly skilled surgeon can still use the technique, but only with extreme caution, by protecting the cornea with viscoelastic substances. To document the preoperative status of the endothelium, specular microscopy should be performed.

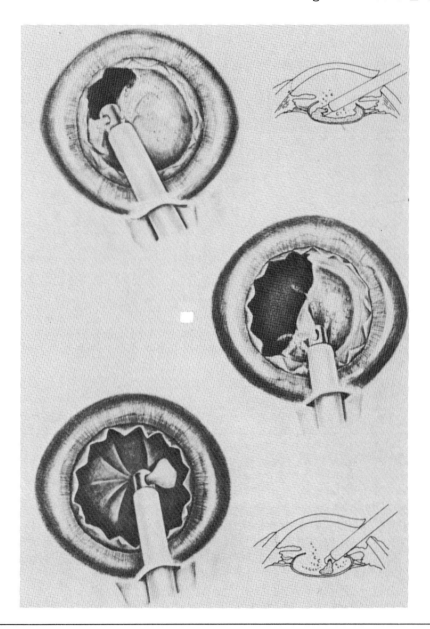

Figure 4.13   ECCE. The cortex is stripped and removed from the eye. (Reprinted with permission from Steele, AD and Drews, RC. Cataract Surgery. Butterworth's International Medical Reviews. London: Butterworth-Heinemann, 1984.)

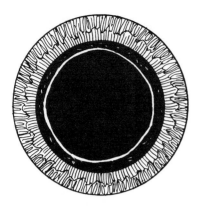

Figure 4.14
Capsulorhexis. A continuous circular tear is made in the anterior capsule using forceps. (Courtesy of Matthew J. Garston, O.D.)

Miotic pupil. Phacoemulsification should not be attempted through a small pupil except by the most experienced surgeons. For patients on chronic miotic therapy for glaucoma, the iris sphincter usually needs to be cut to create a larger pupil and easier access to the cataract. This procedure is termed a *sphincterotomy.*

Subluxed lens. A subluxed, or dislocated, lens is best removed using intracapsular or pars plana vitrectomy techniques.

Phacoemulsification consists of certain basic steps with many subtle variations thereof:

- A 3.5mm to 4.0mm incision is made either at or posterior to the limbus.
- A second opening is sometimes made into the eye at the 2 o'clock position on the limbus. This *stab incision* is just large enough to insert an instrument called a nucleus rotator that will be used to manipulate the nucleus during emulsification and position the IOL once it is inserted in the eye (Figure 4.16).
- The anterior capsulotomy is performed using either the conventional can-opener technique or a newer technique known as *capsulorhexis*, a planned circular tear of the anterior capsule made with forceps (Figure 4.14). The advantages over traditional can-opener techniques include:
  - Less force on the zonules during the procedure, thus less zonular damage
  - The smooth edge of the opening is more resistant to radial tears, seen commonly in the can-opener technique. These tears can extend to the equator of the capsule, resulting in escape of a haptic from the capsular bag and possible lens decentration.
  - Better visibility of the intraocular lens (IOL), allowing for easier lens centration and in-the-bag verification
- The lens nucleus is now ready for emulsification. The instrument used consists of a titanium needle tip that vibrates up to 40,000 times per second. This causes liquifaction of the nucleus, which is then aspirated (removed) from the eye (Figure 4.15). Fluid (balanced salt) is pumped into the eye to take its place.

Figure 4.15
Phacoemulsification of the nucleus
using an ultrasonic instrument.
(Reprinted from Steele, AD and Drews,
RC. Cataract Surgery. Butterworth's
International Medical Reviews.
London: Butterworth-Heinemann,
1984)

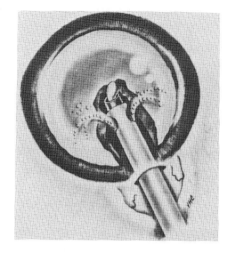

Some surgeons manipulate the nucleus into the anterior chamber, and perform the emulsification there. A more recent trend is to emulsify the nucleus in the posterior chamber, well away from the cornea where endothelial damage can occur (Figure 4.16). Once the nucleus is entirely removed, the phaco instrument and nucleus rotator are removed from the eye.

• Aspiration of cortical material and posterior capsule polishing are now performed, as described in steps 4 and 5 of the section entitled "Planned Extra-capsular Cataract Extraction" earlier in this chapter.

• The small opening made to insert the phaco instrument may need to be enlarged, especially if a conventional rigid lens is to be inserted. If a foldable silicone lens is used, the opening may be adequate. Once the implant is inserted, the wound is closed as will be described later in this chapter.

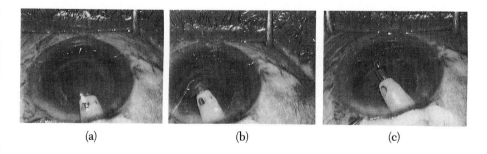

| (a) | (b) | (c) |

Figure 4.16   Phacoemulsification. A tunnel is initially carved out of the
central nucleus (a). The nucleus rotator is used to manipulate
remaining pieces of nucleus toward the phaco instrument (b).
The nucleus is completely emulsified (c) in an average time of
one to two minutes.

	ECCE	Phacoemulsification
Wound size	10–12mm	3.5–6.0mm (depending on type of IOL)
Nucleus	Removed from eye in one piece	Fragmented ultrasonically inside eye and aspirated out
Instrumentation	Basic	More costly, complex
Skill level	Moderate	High

Table 4.1 The Differences between ECCE and Phacoemulsification

The major differences between a conventional planned extracapsular procedure and phacoemulsification are summarized in Table 4.1.

■ INCISION SIZE AND CLOSURE TECHNIQUES

Much attention has been paid to incision size and wound closure techniques. Induced astigmatism, with or against the rule, can be extremely annoying to the patient and sometimes debilitating as well. Even with an otherwise technically successful cataract extraction, if a patient cannot be corrected to a crisp 20/20 postoperatively, they may judge the procedure less than adequate.

The sutures must be tight enough to prevent wound leakage and against-the-rule astigmatism but not so tight as to cause significant irregular or with-the-rule astigmatism. To this end, surgical keratometers were developed and are still used by a few surgeons to monitor wound closure.

□ Intracapsular and Planned Extracapsular Wound Closure

As has been discussed earlier, relatively large limbal incisions are required for conventional ICCE and ECCE. The majority of incisions are closed with 10-0 nonabsorbable nylon sutures, using a variety of techniques. Two of the most common are interrupted (radial) and running (continuous) sutures. There appear to be no distinct advantages of one technique over the other. Interrupted sutures can be removed selectively when trying to reduce astigmatism. Continuous sutures may provide more consistent tension along the wound and less chance of wound gape.

□ Phacoemulsification Wound Closure

The main advantage of phacoemulsification is a small wound. This advantage is somewhat negated when a conventional posterior chamber IOL is inserted, requiring enlargement of the wound to at least 6.0mm. New lenses have been developed, however, that allow the wound size to remain small. Depending on the type of implant used, the incision size itself ranges from 4.0mm to 6.5mm. A 6.5mm silicone lens can be folded and inserted through an incision no larger than 4.0mm. Conventional PMMA lenses, either round or oval, are available in widths ranging from 5.0mm to 7.0mm, requiring the wound to be enlarged to the appropriate size.

When the incision is made at the limbus, unwanted astigmatism can still be induced. A significant advancement in surgical technique involves the use of a scleral pocket incision, 2–4mm behind the limbus, to minimize induced corneal astigmatism (Figure 4.17 and 4.18). These scleral incisions tend to heal faster because of their small size, and often require no sutures. The only disadvantage of posterior scleral incisions is the higher incidence of postoperative hyphema. With few exceptions, these resolve quickly with no permanent damage to the vision or eye (see Chapter 6).

Three commonly used closure techniques for phacoemulsification are:

Conventional limbal closure. A number of surgeons still prefer to use a limbal incision with phacoemulsification, closing the wound with either one or two continuous (X-shaped) or several interrupted sutures. These sutures can induce cylinder as mentioned, and may need to be cut at some point postoperatively.

No-stitch closure. Many patients require no suturing of the small scleral incision. Intraocular pressure creates a self-sealing and very secure wound. The wound is tested for a tight seal and the conjunctiva is brought down over the wound

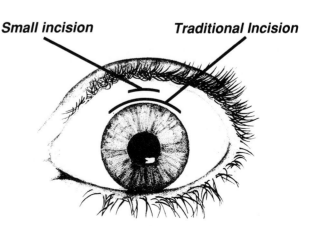

Figure 4.17
A small scleral incision compared to the traditional limbal incision. (Courtesy of Medical Care International.)

Small incision   *Traditional Incision*

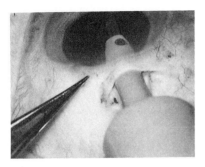

Figure 4.18
A scleral pocket incision 4mm posterior to the limbus (seen here with the phaco unit inserted through it).

and cauterized (Figure 4.19). Postoperatively it can be very difficult to locate the wound site (Figure 4.20).

One-stitch closure. For added safety, some surgeons will put a single 10-0 nylon suture in the scleral wound, either parallel or perpendicular to the horizontal incision (Figure 4.21).

Small incision cataract surgery has received much publicity under the names *one-stitch* and *no-stitch*. Some ophthalmic surgeons have scrambled to learn the new technique for its intrinsic marketing value. Others who have already been doing phacoemulsification for some time see it as a refinement of an already well-proven technique. A major advantage of small incision surgery is better control of the eye *during* the surgery. If a patient moves suddenly or experiences a medical emergency, the surgeon can remove instruments quickly without having to worry about closing a large wound. If this occurs with a large, 12mm incision, complications such as vitreous loss, uveal prolapse, and expulsive hemorrhage are likelier to occur.

A secondary benefit of no-stitch surgery for both surgeon and co-managing doctor of optometry is the elimination of trips back to the surgeon's office for suture cutting. This is a real advantage for people from rural settings who must

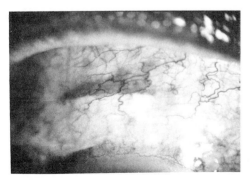

Figure 4.19
A no-stitch scleral incision as seen one week postoperatively.

Figure 4.20
A no-stitch scleral incision can be very difficult to locate, as can be seen in this patient at the four-week postoperative visit.

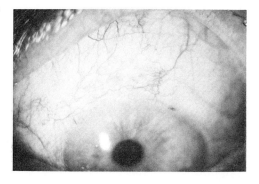

Figure 4.21
A horizontal mattress suture used to secure a scleral pocket incision. (Courtesy of Robert B. Pinkert, OD)

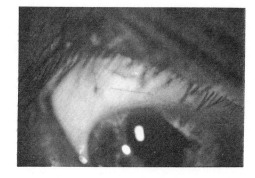

travel some distance for surgery. The added benefits of more rapid healing and a quicker final spectacle prescription are all appreciated by the patient.

☐ Refractive Cataract Surgery

The growing number of surgeons switching to small incision scleral techniques also means that fewer patients will experience induced astigmatism. When there is little or no astigmatism to begin with, the end result is good. When moderate to high astigmatism is present preoperatively, however, the same amount will often be present postoperatively. The cataract surgery is successful, but the astigmatism remains, forcing patients to rely on a distance correction. Refractive cataract surgery is gaining acceptance as an adjunct technique done at the time of cataract extraction and designed to reduce or eliminate preoperative astigmatism. One or two small corneal incisions are made along the steepest meridian, parallel to the limbus and usually outside the 7mm optical zone. Two incisions might be used, for example, in a patient with 3 diopters of cylinder axis 90. One is placed at 3 o'clock and the other is placed 180 degrees away at 9 o'clock. These transverse or relaxing incisions can be very effective in neutralizing this cylinder and may become an integral part of cataract surgery in the future.

□ The Future

At present, surgical technology is advancing so rapidly that even the methods just described may soon be rendered obsolete. YAG laser capsulorhexis and nuclear fragmentation, injectable implants, and other experimental techniques may become the methodology of the future. It is extremely important that the primary care practitioner keep abreast of this rapidly changing technology.

INTRAOCULAR LENS IMPLANTS

□ Indications

Well over one million cataract procedures are performed each year, and the vast majority of patients undergoing surgery are corrected with IOLs. There are three possible methods of aphakic correction: spectacles, contact lenses, and IOLs. The most natural restoration of vision occurs with a lens implant.

In the early years of lens implantation (1975–1980), a great deal of time was spent explaining the advantages of IOLs to patients:

- Less size magnification and optical distortion compared to spectacles or contact lenses
- No restriction of visual field as exists with aphakic spectacles
- Nothing to handle or clean as is necessary with contact lenses

The disadvantages were also discussed: lens instability and decentration, high risk of corneal decompensation, and other possible long-term complications and rejection. The patient was then asked to make a decision, with the guidance of the surgeon.

Today, this situation has changed dramatically. IOLs have been used routinely for over 20 years, and while early lens designs caused a significant number of problems, modern anterior chamber and posterior chamber IOLs are now well tolerated in the majority of cases. When a patient requires cataract surgery, there is usually no need for a lengthy discussion on visual correction alternatives. Unless there are strong contraindications, an IOL is routinely implanted.

Reasons *not* to put an IOL in an eye include:

Young age. Age restrictions for intraocular lens implantation have been relaxed significantly in recent years. In the early 1980s, many surgeons adhered to an unwritten standard of care that did not allow for implants in anyone under age 50. As IOL and surgical technology improved, the age barrier dropped fairly quickly—today most surgeons feel comfortable implanting lenses in any patient over the age of 20. Patients under 20 years of age pose a more difficult dilemma. Lens implants are usually not done on infants and young children with congenital cataracts due to the rapidly changing power of the eye through childhood.

High myopia. High myopes (above 12 diopters) typically do not need an implant because simply removing the cataract will result in a nearly emmetropic eye.

Preexisting ocular disease. Some ocular disease conditions may be contraindications for lens implantation. These include rubeosis irides from proliferative diabetic retinopathy or venous occlusive disease. Chronic uveitis was previously a contraindication and may still be, depending on the severity. Patients with conditions such as Fuch's heterochromic iridocyclitis often do well with a lens implant. Many conditions that used to contraindicate lens implantation such as open angle glaucoma, background diabetic retinopathy, and a blind fellow eye are all compatible with successful IOL surgery. Indications have and will continue to change over time.

□ Selection

LENS DESIGN

The evolution of IOL design is interesting and is briefly summarized here for historical purposes. One of the first IOLs to be used was a posterior chamber lens implanted in London in 1949. Because of its weight, there were significant problems with decentration. Iris-fixated lenses, also known as iris-plane or iris-supported lenses, were developed to improve lens stability by attaching directly to the iris. The most popular of these lenses was the Binkhorst four-loop with two loops in front of the iris and two loops behind the iris holding the lens in place (Figure 4.22). A suture was sometimes placed through the superior haptic and iris to prevent displacement of the lens into the anterior chamber or vitreous (Figure 4.23). The movement of the iris itself was the downfall of this lens, which has not been used since the late 1970s.

Rigid anterior chamber lenses were developed in the 1960s and 1970s but are no longer used because of problems with iris erosion, chronic inflammation, and ocular pain. Today's redesigned, flexible anterior chamber lenses are useful in patients who undergo (or have in the past undergone) an intracapsular extraction (Figure 4.24). These lenses are also commonly used as a secondary implant in aphakes who no longer can or want to wear contact lenses or aphakic spectacles. In time, there will be fewer and fewer patients who do not have a lens implanted at the time of surgery.

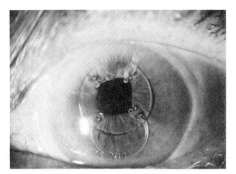

Figure 4.22
Binkhorst four-loop iris-fixated lens.

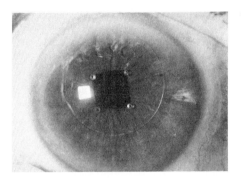

Figure 4.23
A Medallion iris-fixated lens held in place with a superior haptic suture. (Courtesy of Howell Findley, OD)

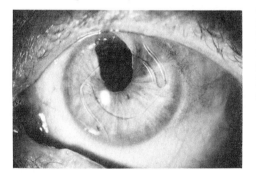

Figure 4.24
Modern anterior chamber lenses, usually reserved for secondary implant procedures, use flexible haptics that prevent movement and decentration.

It is now recognized that the most appropriate place for a lens implant is in the *posterior chamber.* Investigators learned through experience with iris-plane and anterior chamber lenses that the posterior chamber is the most stable and optically accurate location in which to place a lens. Because of its proximity to the nodal point, size magnification is not a factor. Due to the stability of the lens, patients can be widely dilated without fear of dislocation (Figure 4.25). There are many subtle design variations of the basic posterior chamber lens, some of which are shown in Figure 4.26. Lens sizes range from 5.0mm to 7.0mm in diameter (Figure 4.27). The most commonly used size has been 6.0mm, but with the advent of small incision techniques, some surgeons are using a 5.0mm × 6.0mm oval lens.

Figure 4.25
A modern posterior chamber lens is advantageous because of its location and the ability to widely dilate the pupil without fear of subluxation.

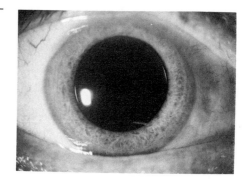

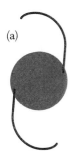
(a)

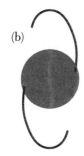
(b)

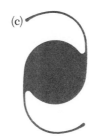
(c)

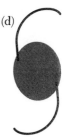
(d)

Figure 4.26   Posterior chamber lenses are available in a wide variety of designs. Shown here are a C-loop multipiece (a), a J-loop multipiece (b), a single piece (c), and a 5.0 × 6.0mm oval (d) lens used in small incision surgery. (Courtesy of Chiron-IntraOptics)

Figure 4.27
A J-loop posterior chamber lens compared in size to a penny.
(Courtesy of Allergan Medical Optics)

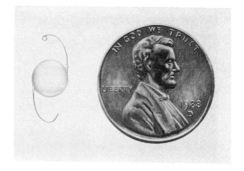

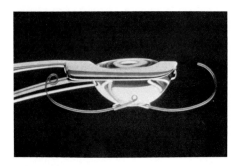

Figure 4.28
A flexible silicone lens seen here folded in half using a special holder/ inserter. (Courtesy of Allergan Medical Optics)

LENS MATERIALS

Most anterior and posterior chamber lenses are made from polymethylmethacrylate (PMMA), the same basic material used in conventional hard contact lenses. Lenses made entirely of PMMA are preferred over older lenses with polypropylene loops because of this material's possible role in postoperative inflammation. The main advantage of the new one-piece PMMA design appears to be better centration. Most PMMA lenses currently manufactured incorporate an ultraviolet (UV) coating. While definitive clinical evidence is lacking, there is enough suspicion of exposure to UV radiation and of its deleterious effects to justify this precaution.

Flexible IOLs made of *silicone* have the advantage of being foldable and thus inserted through a smaller opening (Figure 4.28). Using a special insertion device, the lens then unfolds inside the eye to the size of a conventional posterior chamber lens. The main disadvantage of silicone lenses is that long-term studies regarding stability, optical clarity, and discoloration are lacking.

A significant advancement in optical technology is the *multifocal* IOL. This lens is designed to correct the pseudophakic patient for both distance and near. As with bifocal contact lenses, proper patient selection is critical. Candidates for this lens must clearly understand that their vision may be somewhat compromised at distance and/or near. There are several designs in use, including a diffractive IOL.* All of them require precise surgical centration, minimally induced astigmatism, and emmetropia. These lenses could soon play a major role in the correction of cataract patients.

The use of *hydrogel* intraocular lenses is also under investigation along with other polymers that could possibly be injected into the capsular bag to restore accommodation.

LENS POWER

The appropriate IOL power is chosen by the surgeon after careful keratometry and axial length measurements, which may be provided by the doctor of optom-

---

*While no multifocal lens has been FDA-approved, there are thousands that have been used experimentally.

etry. These measurements, along with the desired postoperative refraction, are put into a lens formula and the IOL power calculated. The desired endpoint is usually emmetropia, but if the fellow eye has already had surgery then an effort should be made to match that refraction. All patients should be told they will need a near correction, and often a minor distance correction, following surgery.

□ Insertion

POSTERIOR CHAMBER LENS

Following removal of the cataract, the next step is insertion of the IOL. The anterior chamber must be well formed and the pupil well dilated during IOL implantation to facilitate entry of the lens into the posterior chamber. One of two methods can be used to accomplish this:

1. *Air* is injected into the anterior chamber in order to keep the chamber deep during IOL insertion. An air bubble is not as effective in protecting the corneal endothelium from trauma but is sometimes used to keep surgical costs down.

2. *Visco-elastic substances* are made from various synthetic and natural compounds. They include Healon (sodium hyaluronate), Viscoat (chondroitin sulfate), and Occucoat (hydroxypropylmethylcellolose). The purpose of injecting this material into the eye before lens insertion is to maintain a deep anterior chamber, protect the corneal endothelium from IOL touch, and expand the capsular bag to allow for easier *in-the-bag* insertion. These substances may not be necessary for every procedure, but they do provide the surgeon a big advantage in difficult cases and when dealing with diseased corneas. The material must be completely aspirated from the eye following IOL insertion to prevent elevation of intraocular pressure.

It may be necessary to enlarge the original incision slightly, depending on the lens type and size. The capsular bag and anterior chamber are filled with air or viscoelastic substance. The IOL is then inserted, using one of the three techniques shown in Figure 4.29. Once the implant is in position, a miotic drug such as carbachol or miochol is injected into the anterior chamber to constrict the pupil and ensure that the IOL will stay in place during the initial 24- to 48-hour recovery period.

In an aphakic individual who can no longer tolerate spectacle or contact lens correction, a secondary IOL is an excellent alternative. If the original surgery was extracapsular, a secondary posterior chamber IOL is most desirable. In cases where the capsule is only partially intact, a secondary posterior chamber lens may still be inserted and attached with sutures through the pars plana. If an intracapsular procedure was performed, an anterior chamber IOL is the lens of choice. If vitreous is present in the anterior chamber, it must be removed before IOL insertion. Viscoelastic substance is then injected into the eye, and the lens is inserted.

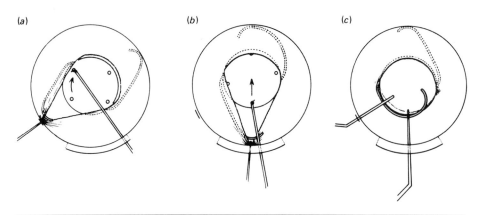

Figure 4.29   Various techniques of IOL insertion including dialing (a), inferior loop compression (b), and superior loop compression (c). (Reprinted with permission of the publisher from Steele, AD and Drews, RC. Cataract Surgery. Butterworth's International Medical Reviews. London: Butterworth-Heinemann, 1984.)

Occasionally, an anterior chamber or iris-fixated lens that has caused corneal decompensation may have to be removed at the same time a corneal transplant is performed. The lens that is removed can usually be replaced with a flexible anterior chamber IOL.

□ Methods of Fixation

Anterior chamber lenses are used as secondary implants or in cases of capsular rupture and unplanned intracapsular surgery. They are fixated by flexible haptics that rest on the iris surface and are held in place by springlike tension (see Figure 4.24).

Posterior chamber lenses are held in place by capsular (in-the-bag) fixation or by ciliary sulcus fixation. It is preferable to place both haptics in the capsular bag (Figure 4.30a). This requires more skill and use of techniques, such as capsulorhexis, that allow the entire anterior capsular edge to be visualized. The advantages of capsular bag fixation include:

Less direct contact of the intraocular lens with surrounding structures. The lens haptics are completely enclosed within the lens capsule, isolating them from the iris and ciliary body.

Less chance of lens decentration. A posterior chamber lens is much less likely to decenter if both haptics are secured within the capsular bag (Figure 4.30b).

Less chance of pupillary capture (see Chapter 6).

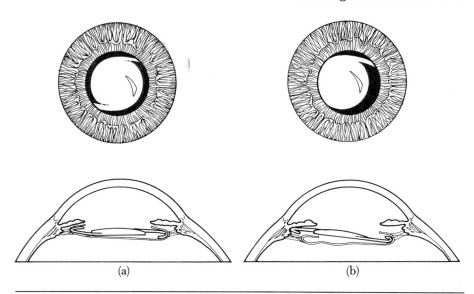

Figure 4.30   Capsular bag fixation (a) results in better lens centration and less damage to the surrounding uveal tissue. One or both haptics out of the bag and in the ciliary sulcus (b) may result in lens decentration. (Courtesy of Matthew J. Garston, O.D.)

INTRAOPERATIVE COMPLICATIONS

Despite the fact that cataract surgery has become a routine procedure, it takes a highly trained surgeon to handle all the challenges that each case presents. A prominent brow can hamper insertion of instruments into the eye. A pupil that will not fully dilate can make cataract removal and lens insertion extremely difficult. A hard nucleus may necessitate prolonged phacoemulsification, which can lead to corneal edema. These potential intraoperative complications and many more are handled routinely by the skilled surgeon, usually without consequence.

Major intraoperative complications are rare and include rupture of the posterior lens capsule, vitreous loss, and expulsive hemorrhage.

□ Rupture of the Lens Capsule

During extracapsular or phacoemulsification surgery, extreme care must be taken not to rupture the posterior capsule while in the process of removing the cortex. A small break in the posterior capsule may not be of any consequence, but a larger break can allow any remaining nuclear material to escape back into the vitreous or vitreous to prolapse forward into the anterior chamber. A significant rupture with vitreous loss may necessitate an anterior vitrectomy and anterior chamber IOL.

□ Vitreous Loss

Vitreous loss is defined as vitreous that prolapses into the anterior chamber and out through the surgical wound. Loss of vitreous during surgery is uncommon if care is taken to leave the posterior capsule intact. The eye must also be soft prior to surgery, using the techniques described, to keep vitreous pressure low and prevent forward movement. The surgeon recognizes increased vitreous pressure clinically when the lens and iris begin to bulge forward during the procedure.

If vitreous does prolapse into the anterior chamber toward the wound, problems may result which include:

- Bullous keratopathy
- Cystoid macular edema
- Chronic anterior uveitis
- Secondary glaucoma
- Vitreous hemorrhage
- Retinal detachment

Initial management involves immediate closure of the wound. The remainder of the case, including lens insertion, may need to be postponed. Once vitreous loss has occurred, surgical removal of the vitreous may be required. If the cornea has decompensated or the retina is detached, surgical management of these problems is also necessary. Uveitis, cystoid macular edema, and glaucoma can usually be managed medically (see Chapter 6).

□ Expulsive Hemorrhage

This disastrous intraoperative complication is fortunately very rare. For unknown reasons, the short posterior ciliary arteries rupture at the time of surgery with forward bowing of the lens and iris. This is followed by the appearance of blood in the anterior chamber with possible extrusion of ocular contents through the wound. An expulsive hemorrhage can also occur within the first few days after surgery, possibly related to a Valsalva's maneuver (increased venous pressure from straining or coughing). Treatment in the case of mild hemorrhage involves careful observation, hopefully with spontaneous clearing. Surgical intervention may be indicated in more serious cases.

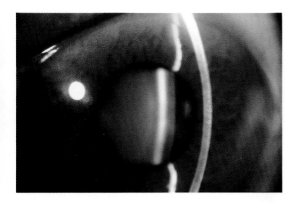

Plate 1 Brunescent nuclear sclerosis.

Plate 2 Milky nuclear sclerosis, giving the appearance of a lens within a lens.

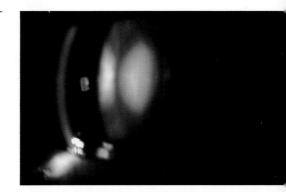

Plate 3 A Morgagnian cataract, showing the nucleus sinking inferiorly within the liquified cortex.

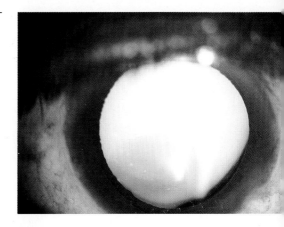

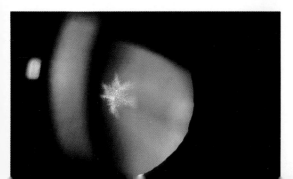

Plate 4 Deposits on the anterior lens capsule from long-term use of Thorazine.

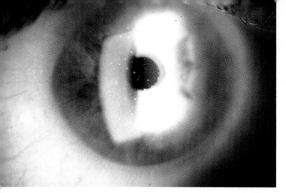

Plate 5 Diffuse stellate keratic precipitates in one eye are often pathognomonic of Fuch's heterochromic iridocyclitis.

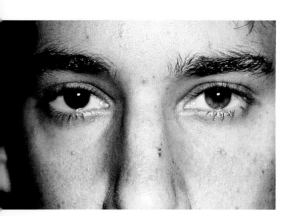

Plate 6 The iris of the involved left eye of this 24-year-old patient is lighter in color than is the right eye because of chronic Fuch's heterochromic iridocyclitis.

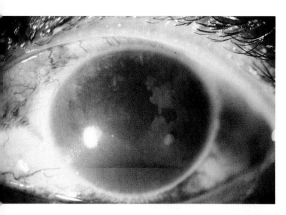

Plate 7 A 15 percent hyphema and large clot on the iris surface, obscuring the pupil. The blood is totally cleared, and the vision is improved to 20/20.

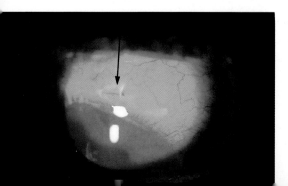

Plate 8 Traumatic wound dehiscence in a 28-year-old male. The patient developed a cataract after a penetrating injury and three weeks after surgery was hit in the eye with a fist, causing a small wound separation (arrow).

Plate 9 Uveal prolapse into the wound 3 days following no-stitch surgery. This 68-year-old woman fell while she was walking her dog and landed directly on her operated eye.

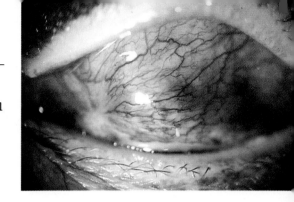

Plate 10 Blood staining of the cornea from a total hyphema associated with elevated intraocular pressure. The patient required a corneal transplant.

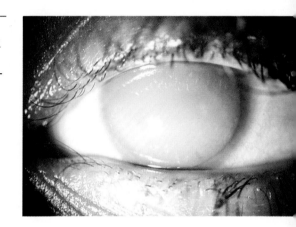

Plate 11 Endophthalmitis in a 67-year-old male who underwent cataract surgery and two days later presented with poor vision and pain. Note the hypopyon in the A/C.

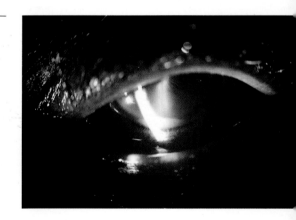

Plate 12 The vitreous inflammation in endophthalmitis is often so severe that it obscures the view of the fundus.

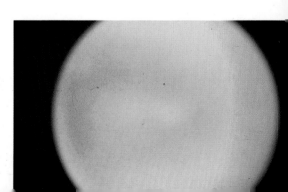

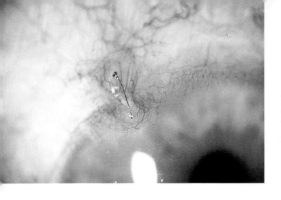

Plate 13 A loose but intact suture with an exposed knot and surrounding inflammatory response.

Plate 14 A localized GPC response (arrow) caused by the loose suture in Plate 13.

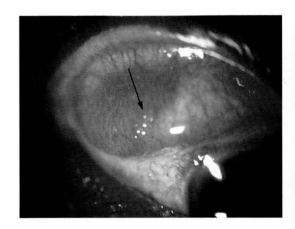

Plate 15 Cystoid macular edema, demonstrating the typical cystic or *honeycomb* appearance.

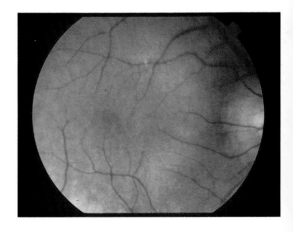

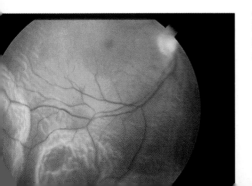

Plate 16 A retinal detachment, noted eighteen months after cataract surgery.

Figure 4.31
Following surgery, the patient's eye is patched, and a protective shield is put in place. The patient is monitored for a short period of time and then released.

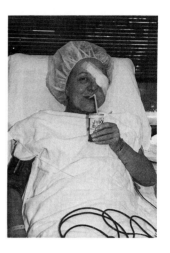

■

PATIENT RECOVERY AND DISCHARGE

Following the procedure, a subconjunctival injection of antibiotic and steroid may be given. The depot steroid injection may be observed by the patient or the family as an alarming white spot on the eye. Reassurance can be given that this is a normal finding and will resolve within several weeks. An antibiotic ointment is instilled, and the eye is patched with a protective shield. Patients are wheeled out to the recovery room and given something to drink (Figure 4.31). Vital signs, such as pulse and blood pressure, are monitored for a short period of time. Once stable, patients are sent home with instructions to resume normal activities if they feel well enough to do so. The only restriction placed on most patients is lifting heavy objects (over 10 pounds). They are given an appointment to be seen the next day at which time further instructions are given and medications started.

5

The Postoperative Evaluation

☐

The doctor of optometry is playing an increasingly important role in the care of the cataract patient once surgery has been performed. Some principles of postoperative cataract care:

- While general guidelines as to normal healing exist, all patients must be considered individually. No two people recover at exactly the same rate.
- Standard follow-up protocol will vary depending on intraoperative or postoperative complications, patient anxiety, level of compliance, and the philosophy of the individual surgeon.
- Instruct patients clearly on proper postoperative care, precautions, and expected visual recovery (Figure 5.1). *Urge them to call you immediately, day or night, in the event of vision loss, pain, or injury to the eye.* Be available to your patients after hours or have a back-up call system in place.
- With each successive visit, improvement of visual acuity and the anterior segment findings should be noted. Any reduction in best corrected acuity or increase in discomfort or inflammation could indicate a problem requiring further investigation.

■
EXAMINATION PROTOCOL

☐ Follow-up Schedule

The number of postoperative visits, the interval between visits, and which doctor sees the patient on a given visit are usually determined by the surgeon. A co-management schedule followed by many progressive practitioners is summarized in Table 5.1. The number of visits may, of course, be increased or decreased depending on the individual rate of healing and the presence of complications. In the event of a serious problem such as endophthalmitis or a wound leak, the surgeon may justifiably elect to do most of the follow-up. The doctor of optometry should be kept closely informed in these cases to enable intelligent communication with the patient and the patient's family.

POST OPERATIVE SCHEDULE
Please Read Carefully!

Medication Schedule

You will be using <u>two</u> different **eye drops** beginning the day after your surgery.

The first drop, Genoptic, is an antibiotic and the same one you used 3 days before your surgery. It is a <u>clear drop</u>, and is to be used in your operated eye **4** times a day for **one** week only. After one week you may stop this drop.

The second eyedrop, Pred Forte, is a steroid to decrease inflammation. It is a <u>milky drop</u>, and is to be used as follows:

4 times a day for the first week
3 times a day for the second week
2 times a day for the third week
1 time a day for the fourth week

It should be stopped after 4 weeks unless your doctor instructs you differently.

Eye Shield

Please wear the plastic eye shield given to you at the completion of your surgery every night for the **4** weeks following surgery. This is <u>very</u> important, and is for your own protection!!! You will not need to wear the shield during the day, but glasses or sunglasses should be worn for protection.

Postoperative Care

Your eye doctor will need to see you at regular intervals to be sure your eye is healing properly. You should be sure and keep the following appointed schedule with your family eye doctor.

Visit #1	1 week after surgery
Visit #2	4 weeks after surgery
Visit #3	8 weeks after surgery

Six Month Postoperative Visit

You will also need to see your eye doctor at approximately six months after you have had cataract surgery. You may need a final change in your spectacle correction at that time. In addition, you may then be ready to consider cataract surgery in your other eye. Your eye doctor can tell you if cataract surgery would benefit your other eye at that time.

If you encounter any pain or sudden change in vision in your operated eye, contact your eye doctor or Omni Eye Services <u>immediately</u>.

The doctors and staff at Omni Eye Services certainly appreciate the opportunity to have assisted you in regaining your sight and wish you a safe, speedy recovery.

The Omni Eye Services Staff

Figure 5.1 Postoperative instructions regarding medication, follow-up schedule, and eye protection are extremely important.

Visit Number	Time after Surgery	Doctor Seen
1	1 day	Surgeon
2	1 week	Surgeon or Doctor of Optometry
3	3–4 weeks	Doctor of Optometry
4	6–8 weeks	Doctor of Optometry
5	4–6 months	Doctor of Optometry

Table 5.1   A Typical Schedule of Postoperative Co-management between the Ophthalmic Surgeon and the Doctor of Optometry

□ Postoperative Medications

On the one day postoperative visit, the patient will be placed on a topical antibiotic to prevent infection and given a topical steroid to reduce the anterior chamber inflammation. Some surgeons prescribe a steroid-antibiotic combination drop for patient convenience. Others prefer a separate antibiotic and steroid so the drugs can be tapered individually. Depending on the surgeon and the surgical result, the specific topical medications and dosage will vary. The most commonly used medications are listed in Table 5.2. Two frequently used postoperative medication schedules are outlined in Table 5.3.

The steroid dosage may require modification due to a number of factors:

Persistent or rebound iritis. If the anterior chamber reaction (cell and flare) does not subside as expected, the patient may require a higher dosage for a longer period of time. If cell and flare recur after the steroid is discontinued, the drop should be restarted and tapered more slowly.

Cylinder. Some surgeons will adjust the dosage of topical steroid in an attempt to control postoperative astigmatism. By delaying wound healing, topical steroids can in some cases reduce with-the-rule astigmatism.

Antibiotics	Steroids	Steroid-Antibiotic Combinations
Gentamicin	Pred Forte	Pred-G
Tobramycin	Inflammase Forte	Tobradex
Polytrim	FML Forte	Maxitrol
Ciloxan		Neo Decadron

Table 5.2   Commonly Used Medications for the Postoperative Cataract Patient

Topical antibiotic
  1 drop QID × 1 Week
  then discontinue
Prednisolone 1% (Phosphate or Acetate)
  1 drop QID for 1st Week
  1 drop TID for 2nd Week
  1 drop BID for 3rd Week
  1 drop QD for 4th Week
  then discontinue

OR:

Topical steroid-antibiotic combination (i.e. Pred-G)
  1 drop QID for 1st Week
  1 drop TID for 2nd Week
  1 drop BID for 3rd Week
  1 drop QD for 4th Week
  then discontinue

Table 5.3 Two Common Postoperative Medication Schedules. There Are Many Variations to This, Depending on Surgeon Preference.

Steroid responder. Only rarely will a patient develop elevated IOP (intraocular pressure) from the topical steroid. This response may be difficult to distinguish from a pressure rise secondary to inflammatory debris in the trabeculum. If suspicion of steroid-induced glaucoma exists, there are several management options:

1. Continue the steroid and add an antiglaucoma medication (such as a beta blocker) twice a day.

2. Switch to a different steroid such as FML Forte. This medication seems to induce less elevation of pressure while maintaining good anti-inflammatory activity.

3. Try a topical nonsteroidal anti-inflammatory agent such as Voltaren (diclofenac sodium). This medication is approved for use in treating postsurgical iritis and does not seem to affect intraocular pressure as steroids can.

□ Protecting the Eye

Patients should be counseled on the importance of protecting the operated eye. Certain precautions will help prevent blunt trauma to the eye that could lead to wound dehiscence or other complications:

Procedure	Visit				
	1 day	1 week	3–4 weeks	6–8 weeks	4–6 months
Case history	X	X	X	X	X
VA	X	X	X	X	X
Refraction		*	X	X	*
Keratometry			X	*	*
Gross external exam	X	X	X		
Neuroscreen					X(**)
Slit lamp	X	X	X	X	X
Tonometry	X	X	X	X	X
Dilated fundus exam				*	X(**)

X = To be done at specified visit
* = Optional/if needed
** = To be done sooner if patient presents with vision or field loss

Table 5.4   A Suggested Schedule of Postoperative Examination Procedures

- Spectacle lenses or sun-shields worn daily as protection
- Protective shield taped over the operated eye at bedtime for three to four weeks to prevent inadvertent injury while sleeping
- Avoid rubbing the operated eye
- No heavy lifting (over ten pounds) for several weeks after surgery. Bending over or straining should be avoided early on in conventional extracapsular surgery. This restriction is usually not placed on patients undergoing small incision procedures.

Activities involving use of the eyes, such as reading or watching TV, should be encouraged.

☐ Postoperative Examination Procedures

Assuming that the surgeon has good technical skills and consistent results, postoperative examinations are usually straightforward and do not require a great deal of time. There are a minimum number of procedures that should be performed at each visit as outlined in Table 5.4. This is only a suggested guideline and will vary depending on the recovery rate of each individual. The components of the postoperative examination are:

CASE HISTORY

- Begin by summarizing the surgical procedure, the eye involved, and the date performed.

Example: S/P ECCE/PC IOL OS 6/9/92

(S/P is an abbreviation for *status post,* meaning the patient has a history of surgery or other events to the eye—for example, S/P hyphema OS, S/P pterygium resection OD, S/P trauma OS.)
• Note which postoperative visit this is.

Example: S/P Phaco/PC IOL OD 6/9/92
(4-week PO visit)

• Ask the patient, "How does your eye feel?" and "How is your vision?" Responses to these questions at the first few postoperative visits might include:
  ○ No problems
  ○ Blurred vision
  ○ Foreign body sensation
  ○ Pain
  ○ Discharge, tearing
  ○ Flashes of light
  ○ Floaters
• Ask about their postoperative medications. Monitor compliance by asking them to bring the drops with them to each visit.

The completed history should look similar to that shown in Figure 5.2.

VISUAL ACUITY AND REFRACTION

Visual acuity (VA) should be checked each time the patient is seen, whether it is a scheduled postoperative visit or an emergency. Check VA before any other testing is done and before instilling drops. Pinhole acuity is helpful in determining the potential for improvement. *Visual acuity should steadily improve with each postoperative visit.* A guide to assessing the patient's visual and refractive status can be found in Table 5.5.

KERATOMETRY

K readings can be taken as baseline beginning at the one-week visit. These readings can assist the practitioner with the refraction if the retinoscopy reflex is poor. With limbal incisions, two to four diopters of *with-the-rule cylinder* is not unusual at one week. A progressive reduction of the cylinder toward plano should be noted over the next six to eight weeks. If the cylinder persists after this time, sutures can be cut to reduce it. If the patient shows *against-the-rule cylinder* postoper-

Figure 5.2
Example of a
postoperative history.

DATE 42 WF S/P Phaco/IOL OS 9/1/92 (1WK PO)
CC: Slight foreign body sensation OS
Meds: Pred Forte 1% OS TID

Visit	Suggested Testing	Expected Acuity
1 Day	Unaided VA + pinhole only	20/30 to 20/200
1 Week	Unaided VA + pinhole	20/20 to 20/80
	Quick refraction for baseline (optional)	
3–4 Weeks	Unaided VA + refraction (some one-stitch/no-stitch patients ready for final prescription [Rx])	20/20 to 20/40
6–8 Weeks	Unaided VA + refraction (most patients ready for final Rx)	20/20
4–6 Months	Aided VA; if not 20/20, re-refraction/modification; If not correctable to 20/20, look for cause	20/20

Note: These acuities are estimates of what is usually seen in a successful surgical case, not absolute findings. Depending on postoperative complications and the status of the fundus, acuity can range from 20/20 to light perception only at any given visit.

Table 5.5 Guide for Assessing Visual/Refractive Status

atively that was not present before surgery, notify the surgeon. This indicates a possible wound separation that may need resuturing. Look for a positive Seidel sign (Figure 5.3).

NEURO-OCULAR SCREENING

Confrontation visual fields, motility, and pupillary testing may become necessary if there is any evidence of postoperative vision loss or diplopia from an ischemic event or neurological complication. These tests should probably be performed routinely at the four to six month visit.

GROSS EXTERNAL EXAMINATION

Prior to the slit lamp examination, a gross external view of the eyelids and globe is necessary to determine the presence of swelling, ptosis, bruises, and the pattern of bulbar injection:

Lids. Look for ptosis. Occasionally the lid will be swollen and give the appearance of ptosis, but it is actually a pseudoptosis that resolves with the swelling. True ptosis can follow cataract surgery (see Chapter 6), and should be documented by measuring the interpalpebral fissures of both eyes. Bruises (ecchymosis) of the lids or skin surrounding the lids may be seen and should be documented.

Bulbar conjunctiva. It is often easier to assess the degree and distribution of conjunctival injection and subconjunctival hemorrhages by having the patient look up, down, left, and right prior to the slit lamp exam.

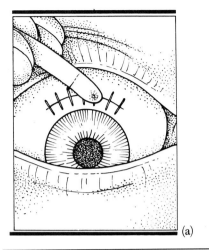 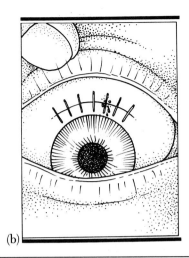

(a)   (b)

Figure 5.3   The Seidel Test. "Paint" a wet fluorescein strip over the area of
the wound (a) and look for a dark stream of fluid (aqueous) or
bubbles interrupting the green dye (b). This is referred to as a
positive Seidel sign. (Reprinted with permission of the publisher
from Fingeret, M, Casser, L and Woodcome, T. *Atlas of primary
eyecare procedures.* Norwalk, Conn.: Appleton & Lange.)

SLIT LAMP EXAMINATION

The slit lamp examination should be thorough and methodical, looking at each
structure in the same order in every patient. Below is a brief guide of what to
look for at each postoperative visit. Complications are dealt with in more detail
in Chapter 6.

Wound
The wound should be well sealed and the sutures intact and buried. Look carefully
for any separation or rupture of the wound as evidenced by broken sutures or
uveal prolapse. A Seidel test can be used to confirm a wound leak (Figure 5.3).

Cornea
The cornea should be relatively clear, but some degree of trauma to one or more
layers is not uncommon. The clinician should carefully evaluate any changes in
the epithelium, stroma, Descemet's membrane, and endothelium. Specular reflection can be used to estimate the endothelial cell population and compare it
to preoperative counts.

Anterior Chamber (A/C)
It is extremely important to evaluate:

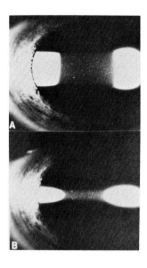

Figure 5.4
For a better view of cell and flare, increase the slit beam's vertical dimension (a) rather than using the conventional conical beam (b).

Depth. The A/C should be deep and well formed. A shallow A/C may indicate a wound leak or possible pupillary block glaucoma. Gonioscopy is often necessary to determine if the angle itself is open.

Cell and flare. Monitoring the degree of cell and flare is the best way to evaluate postoperative inflammation and healing. The cell and flare should be graded separately, using the brightest illumination setting of the slit lamp and a totally darkened room. The slit lamp beam should be opened vertically to enable the examiner to view the cell and flare more easily (Figure 5.4). Postoperative patients usually show more cell than flare, in part due to lenticular debris and pigment that accentuate the inflammatory response. Assuming an uneventful surgical procedure, a typical amount of cell and flare might be:

Day 1. 2–3+ cell/1+ flare

Week 1. 1–2+ cell/trace flare

Week 4. Trace–1+ cell/no flare

Week 8. A/C deep and quiet

Hypopyon. Pus that settles inferiorly in the A/C is referred to as a hypopyon (Plate 11). This is a serious warning sign of bacterial endophthalmitis, an intra-ocular infection after surgery (see Chapter 6). It may simply represent a severe inflammatory response, known as a sterile hypopyon, consisting of white blood cells and fibrin.

Hyphema. An accumulation of blood in the A/C is called a hyphema. It is seen occasionally following planned extracapsular extraction and more commonly after phacoemulsification through a scleral incision. It is most commonly caused by blunt trauma to the eye unrelated to surgery. In its mildest form, red blood cells are suspended in the A/C and condensed on the corneal endothelium in

Figure 5.5
A 25 percent hyphema noted one day
after no-stitch phacoemulsification
surgery.

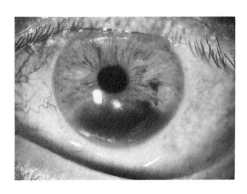

a vertical spindle. Clots may also form on the endothelium or iris surface, with possible obscuration of vision if on the visual axis (Plate 7). When the blood settles inferiorly, the percentage of the A/C it occupies should be estimated and recorded. For example, a 25 percent hyphema indicates that one-quarter of the A/C is filled with blood (Figure 5.5). The patient's most recent head position will often determine whether the blood is settled or scattered throughout the A/C.

Lenticular and iris debris. The A/C should be examined for cortical debris or other remnants of the lens that have not been removed. Loosened pigment from the iris may also be noted.

Vitreous. Vitreous is commonly seen in the anterior chamber following intracapsular surgery. It may also be seen with extracapsular techniques if the posterior capsule is accidentally broken. Once it is noted, look for an intact versus ruptured anterior hyaloid face (AHF) in the A/C. An intact vitreous face that contacts the corneal endothelium has a much greater chance of damaging the cornea (bullous keratopathy) than does a ruptured AHF with loose vitreous in the A/C.

Iris
The iris should look exactly as it did before surgery. Note any displacement or irregularity of the pupil. Except for the one-day visit, the pupil should react normally to direct light without an afferent defect. Note any areas of iris atrophy or transillumination.

Posterior Chamber (P/C) IOL
Look for:

Centered versus decentered position. This may be difficult to determine accurately until the patient is dilated at the six- to eight-week visit.

In-the-bag versus out-of-the-bag status. Look for the anterior edge of the cut capsule *in front of* the IOL to confirm in-the-bag status.

Precipitates or pigment on IOL surface.

Synechia of posterior iris to anterior surface of P/C IOL.

Anterior Chamber IOL
Look for:

Position of implant haptics. (that is, in the angle or touching the endothelium).

Precipitates or pigment on IOL surface.

Posterior Capsule
In a planned extracapsular procedure, the capsule should be fully intact, clear, and without significant folds. Retroillumination is extremely useful in viewing any opacities or tears.

INTRAOCULAR PRESSURE

Goldmann applanation tonometry should be performed at every visit. Intraocular pressure that is either abnormally low (below 6) or high (above 22) may signal complications. Low pressure requires a more careful look at the wound and fundus to rule out dehiscence or choroidal detachment. High pressure may be secondary to inflammatory or lenticular debris in the trabeculum, incomplete removal of viscoelastic material, steroid response, or pupillary block.

FUNDUS EXAMINATION

As mentioned previously, a dilated fundus examination is not necessary at each visit. To be thorough, one might consider dilating the eye at the six- to eight-week visit and again at the four- to six-month visit. Dilation should be performed **immediately** if the patient presents at any time with unexplained vision loss, flashes, or floaters. Attention should be given to the clarity of the vitreous, health of the optic nerve, and integrity of the macula and retinal periphery. A red reflex using the direct ophthalmoscope or retinoscope indicates clear media and a normal healing process.

□ Normal Postoperative Healing

With experience, the co-managing doctor of optometry will become familiar with the individual surgeon's techniques, protocol, and normal course of healing. If a patient is not progressing as expected, the surgeon should always be notified. Always err on the side of caution by seeing patients who complain of vision loss, photopsias, discomfort, or pain *without delay.* Do not hesitate to see them back more frequently than the prescribed follow-up regimen dictates. Follow the rules of sound practice by carefully observing and meticulously recording all examination findings. By doing so, postoperative care of the cataract patient can be extremely rewarding and enjoyable for patient and doctor alike.

6

Diagnosis and Management
of Postoperative
Complications

☐

Complications following cataract surgery are relatively rare in the hands of a competent, experienced surgeon. Some complications such as rebound iritis, elevated intraocular pressure, or induced astigmatism are easily managed. Others, such as endophthalmitis, cystoid macular edema, or retinal detachment, require more involved medical or surgical intervention. This chapter will first deal with the most common complications of cataract surgery (see Table 6.1) and then with complications specific to intraocular lens (IOL) implantation.

■
COMPLICATIONS OF CATARACT SURGERY

Most postoperative complications can be diagnosed accurately by paying careful attention to patient symptoms, time of onset after surgery, and objective ocular findings. Symptoms and possible corresponding complications are summarized in Table 6.2.

☐ Early Complications

EYELIDS

Ptosis
Some degree of lid edema and pseudoptosis may be noted following surgery. As the lid edema resolves, the upper lid is restored to its original configuration. Patients should be reassured of this as they are most often disturbed by the cosmetic appearance of the eye.

Early Complications		Late Complications

Eyelids
  Ptosis
  Ecchymosis
	Cornea
	  Basement membrane changes
	  Epithelial abrasions
	  Superficial punctate keratitis
		High astigmatism

Conjunctiva
  Injection/
    subconjunctival
    hemorrhage
  Chemosis
	Corneal edema
	  Descemet's membrane
	    detachment
	  Endothelial deposits
		Loose sutures/GPC
		
		Bullous keratopathy
		
		Epithelial downgrowth

Extraocular muscles
  Strabismus
	Intraocular Pressure
	  Elevation
	  Hypotony
		Rebound iritis

Operative Wound
  High astigmatism
  Wound leak/
    dehiscence
	Anterior Chamber
	  Hyphema
	  Endophthalmitis
	  Shallow chamber
		Posterior capsular
		  opacification

	Iris
	  Atrophy
	  Mydriasis
	  Distortion
		Cystoid macular
		  edema
		
		Retinal detachment

Table 6.1 Postoperative Complications of Cataract Surgery

The lid speculum or the bridle suture used during surgery may at times cause damage to the levator muscle, resulting in true postoperative ptosis. For this reason, some surgeons are abandoning the use of the bridle suture. The ptosis usually resolves in several months, but surgical repair may become necessary if it persists.

Ecchymosis
Bruises of the upper and lower lid and/or the skin surrounding the lids can occur from either the lid speculum or administration of anesthesia. These bruises will resolve on their own in several weeks without sequelae.

CONJUNCTIVA

Conjunctival Injection
Diffuse or sector bulbar conjunctival and episcleral injection is normal in postoperative cataract patients (Figure 6.1).

Subconjunctival Hemorrhage
Subconjunctival hemorrhages are often seen over the wound although the blood can dissect under a larger area of the conjunctiva. This may lead to a rather

Symptom	Diagnosis Onset after Surgery	
	Early	**Late**
Visual disturbance		
Vision loss	Corneal edema	Cystoid macular edema
	Hyphema	Bullous keratopathy
	Wound leak/choroidal detachment	Capsular opacification
		Retinal detachment
	Endophthalmitis	
Flashes/floaters	Retinal tear/detachment	Retinal tear/detachment
	Posterior vitreous detachment	Posterior vitreous detachment
Monocular ghost images/glare	Induced astigmatism	Displaced IOL
		Uncorrected astigmatism
Diplopia	Retrobulbar injection	Possible nerve palsy
Discomfort/pain		
Foreign body sensation/ irritation	Normal wound sensitivity	Loose suture, exposed suture tip
	Epithelial basement membrane changes	Early corneal decompensation
	Punctate keratitis	
Significant pain	Epithelial abrasion	Pupillary block
	Acute IOP elevation/ pupillary block	Bullous keratopathy
	Endophthalmitis	
Photophobia	Normal A/C inflammation	Rebound iritis
	Corneal edema	Bullous keratopathy

Table 6.2   Etiology of Postoperative Symptoms

Figure 6.1
Sector conjunctival injection and
subconjunctival hemorrhages are a
normal postoperative finding.

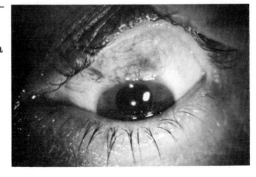

dramatic appearance that is out of proportion to the severity of the problem. Reassurance should be given that the blood will clear within one to two weeks.

Chemosis

Conjunctival chemosis is defined as swelling or ballooning of the conjunctiva in response to trauma, allergy, or infection. Occasionally seen in the postoperative cataract patient, chemosis can be cosmetically disturbing. It may cause corneal exposure due to lid override, resulting in exposure keratitis and possibly dellen formation. Management includes vasoconstrictors and cold compresses for the chemosis and lubricants for the keratitis.

EXTRAOCULAR MUSCLES

Damage to the extraocular muscles can cause postoperative diplopia. Often this acquired diplopia is vertical and is the source of considerable frustration to patient and surgeon alike. Once neurological disorders are ruled out, local restrictive myopathy must be considered. An increasingly recognized problem related to retrobulbar anesthesia is contracture of the inferior rectus muscle, resulting in restricted upgaze. Strabismus surgery may become necessary if these problems do not resolve on their own.

OPERATIVE WOUND

There are several early complications related to the wound that range from annoying to serious.

High Astigmatism

Whenever an incision is made along the limbus, wound closure will invariably induce a certain amount of corneal astigmatism. As a general rule, a moderate amount of *with-the-rule* cylinder—1.5 to 3.0 diopters—is acceptable immediately after surgery. This will usually decrease on its own over time as in this example:

Day 1 $+1.00 = -2.50 \times 180$

Week 3 $+0.50 = -1.00 \times 180$

Week 8 $\text{PLANO} = -0.50 \times 180$

If the induced astigmatic error is greater than 3 diopters, sutures may eventually need to be cut. This is usually recommended at the 8 week visit.

Against-the-rule astigmatism not present preoperatively indicates that the limbal incision was not sutured tightly enough. This may signal an existing or impending wound leak.

As more and more surgeons use small scleral incision techniques, little or no astigmatism is being iatrogenically induced.

Wound Leak/Dehiscence

In addition to against-the-rule astigmatism, other clinical signs of a possible wound leak or dehiscence (separation) include:

- Shallow or flat anterior chamber
- Positive Seidel sign
- Hypotony—IOP (intraocular pressure) below 6mm Hg
- Bleb formation
- Iris prolapse into the wound
- Pupil displaced toward the wound
- Choroidal detachment
- Endopththalmitis

A wound leak may occur spontaneously as a result of inadequate closure and suturing. Wound dehiscence is usually secondary to blunt trauma such as from an accidental fall or a blow to the eye (Plate 8). Excessive straining can result in a sudden elevation of venous pressure, termed a Valsalva's maneuver, which can also separate the wound. These maneuvers include excessive coughing, lifting, or sexual activity.

Suspicion of a wound leak is often confirmed clinically by a shallow anterior chamber (A/C) and positive Seidel sign. A conjunctival bleb will form over the wound as aqueous percolates through the opening in the sclera. IOP may be so low as to be immeasurable. A *choroidal detachment* in the area of the pars plana may rarely accompany a wound leak. The characteristic appearance is that of grayish elevations in the periphery that can be confused with a retinal detachment or mass lesion. Uveal tissue, especially iris, in the wound site is a confirmatory sign of a dehiscence (Plate 9).

Once a wound leak or dehiscence is detected, the surgeon should be notified. If the leak is small, initial management is conservative and consists of simple observation or tight pressure patching for 24 to 48 hours. If a large gape exists, resuturing is indicated. If uveal prolapse accompanies the wound dehiscence, it must be surgically repaired by replacing as much of the iris as possible back into the eye and cutting out the rest. Occasionally, more involved surgery is indicated such as reforming the A/C with air and draining the fluid in the suprachoroidal space. Although most wound problems occur within the first few postoperative months, traumatic wound dehiscence has been observed up to one year after surgery.

CORNEA

During the first two to three weeks of postoperative recovery, minor corneal complications can be seen which are usually self-limiting.

Epithelial Basement Membrane Changes

Stress on the cornea *during* surgery combined with a tightly patched eye *after* surgery can result in minor epithelial basement membrane changes. Often seen superiorly, these changes usually take the form of maps although dots and fingerprints can also be seen. Treatment is seldom necessary, but hypertonic saline can be used if the patient is symptomatic with a foreign-body sensation.

Epithelial Abrasions

Only rarely will a patient present after surgery with an abrasion of the corneal epithelium. Large abrasions should be patched (after instilling an antibiotic ointment) for 24 hours. Small abrasions will heal quickly using topical antibiotics alone. If the defect persists or is irregular in shape, test corneal sensitivity and be suspicious of possible herpetic keratitis.

Superficial Punctate Keratitis

Superficial punctate keratitis (SPK) following surgery is not a normal finding and should be documented. Possible causes include:

Allergic/toxic response to medication. Depending on which topical medications are used postoperatively and for how long, an allergic or toxic response to the cornea can result. The SPK is usually diffuse, which is helpful in differentiating it from bacterial or exposure keratitis. Being alert to medication reactions will enable the practitioner to discontinue or change them in a timely manner.

Exposure. An area of conjunctival chemosis or bleb from a wound leak can cause a lid surfacing abnormality or possible lagophthalmos, resulting in corneal dessication. Lubricant therapy in conjunction with treatment of the underlying problem should eliminate the keratitis.

Corneal Edema

Epithelial microcysts or stromal folds (Figures 6.8 and 6.9a) may be present at the one-day visit, indicative of transient corneal edema. This is usually due to either minor surgical trauma, hypoxia from a tight patch, or elevated IOP. Vision may be somewhat impaired as a result but should clear rapidly within several weeks. Treatment is not necessary unless the underlying cause is high IOP.

Persistent epithelial or stromal edema may indicate more significant damage to the endothelium, and can lead to bullous keratopathy as will be discussed later in this chapter.

Descemet's Membrane Detachment

Very rarely, Descemet's membrane will be inadvertently stripped from the overlying stroma during surgery. This can result in localized endothelial cell dysfunction and eventual corneal edema. If the detachment is large enough, surgery, using air in the A/C, may be necessary to reattach the membrane.

Endothelial Deposits

Loosened iris pigment, inflammatory precipitates, and viscoelastic substances used to protect the endothelium during surgery can all be responsible for deposits on the endothelium. Typically, these will resolve on their own or with the help of a topical steroid.

Figure 6.2
Pupillary block glaucoma in a
patient who underwent
secondary A/C lens implantation
without an iridectomy.

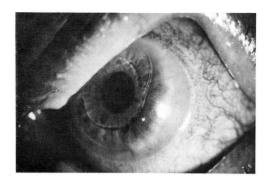

INTRAOCULAR PRESSURE

Elevated Intraocular Pressure (Open Angle)

An increase in IOP following cataract surgery is not uncommon and is usually related to the inflammatory response in the A/C. If the pressure is only moderately increased (22–30mm Hg), treating the inflammation alone with a topical steroid should be sufficient to lower it. An intraocular pressure higher than 30mm Hg should probably be treated with a beta blocker such as Timoptic or Betagan unless medically contraindicated. If the IOP increases to 40 to 50, patients will usually present with a painful eye soon after surgery. Diffuse microcystic edema of the corneal epithelium is often noted. These cases may be related to incomplete removal of viscoelastic substances from the A/C, causing blockage of the trabeculum. The surgeon should be notified, and the patient started on a topical beta blocker. Oral carbonic anhydrase inhibitors are often used as well.

In a patient with a deep chamber and an open angle, other possible causes of elevated IOP following surgery include:

* Topical steroid responder
* Blood in the anterior chamber (hyphema)
* Retained cortical material and lenticular debris
* Tightly sutured wound

Elevated Intraocular Pressure (Closed Angle)

The most common cause of a narrow or closed angle postoperatively is pupillary block. This is usually seen with A/C lenses *without* an iridectomy.

The optic of the implant can cover the pupil in such a way that aqueous has no way of entering the anterior chamber. Iris bombe and a shallow chamber result, along with significant elevation in intraocular pressure (Figure 6.2). Immediate first aid attempts should be made to dilate the pupil beyond the implant, which will alleviate the block. An argon or YAG iridotomy should then be performed to restore aqueous flow and ensure that the pupillary block will not recur. This problem can be avoided if the surgeon does an iridectomy at the time of the implant surgery.

Low Intraocular Pressure (Hypotony)

Wound leaks, as were discussed previously, are usually responsible for low IOP. Other conditions that can create low pressure in a postoperative eye are:

- Inadvertent filtering bleb
- Cyclodialysis cleft
- Ciliary shutdown secondary to severe inflammation
- Choroidal detachment
- Retinal detachment

ANTERIOR CHAMBER

Hyphema

Hyphemas are not common in the postoperative cataract patient. As the trend in surgery shifts toward posterior (away from the limbus) scleral incisions, however, hyphemas are seen more frequently because of the vascularity of the scleral bed.

A hyphema usually takes the form of small clots on the corneal endothelium or the iris surface or layered blood in the inferior A/C (see Plate 7). Visual acuity (VA) is reduced only in the case of an extremely turbid A/C or when a dense clot is located on the visual axis.

Although it is annoying to the surgeon and alarming to the patient, postoperative hyphemas will usually resolve without treatment in a few days to several weeks. The co-managing doctor of optometry should monitor these patients regularly by checking acuity and IOP, and by documenting the appearance of the blood at each visit. Patients should be encouraged to keep their heads elevated and to limit strenuous activity, and they should be reassured that the vision will improve rapidly. If the blood occupies more than 40 percent of the A/C, notify the surgeon, and monitor the intraocular pressure carefully. In cases where the entire chamber is filled with blood and the intraocular pressure is high, the cornea can become permanently blood stained (Plate 10). This can be prevented if it is promptly detected and if the blood is surgically removed from the A/C.

Endophthalmitis

One of the most feared and devastating complications of cataract surgery today is endophthalmitis. This intraocular bacterial infection usually occurs within the first two or three days after surgery, although delayed infections associated with certain organisms or wound leaks can be seen several years postoperatively. Endophthalmitis occurs because of the introduction of pathogenic bacteria into the eye at the time of surgery. The most common organisms responsible for endophthalmitis are listed in Table 6.3. Often the source of infection is unknown, but possible causes include:

- Normal bacterial flora of the conjunctiva
- Nonsterile instruments
- Contaminated solutions (saline or viscoelastics)
- Contaminated intraocular lenses (IOLs)

Organism	Approximate Incidence (percent)
Gram-positive species:	
Staphylococcus epidermidis	40
Staphylococcus aureus	20
Streptococcus species	10
Gram-negative species (including Pseudomonas and Haemophilus)	15
Fungi, propionobacterium, miscellaneous	15

Table 6.3 Most Common Organisms Responsible for Endophthalmitis (Modified from Driebe WT, Mandlebaum S, Forster RK, et al. Pseudophakic endophthalmitis. *Ophthalmology* 1986; 93:442.)

The overall incidence of postoperative endophthalmitis is estimated at one in 2000–3000 cases. The clinical presentation is:

Patient symptoms:

- Moderate to severe ocular pain
- Rapid loss of vision (*Example:* A drop from 20/40 to hand motion within a day)

Clinical signs:

- Lid swelling
- Bulbar conjunctival injection
- Corneal edema (haze and/or folds)
- Severe A/C reaction
- Hypopyon (Plate 11)
- Vitritis with poor or no view of fundus (Plate 12)

It can be difficult to distinguish endophthalmitis from a sterile inflammatory response. If the surgical case was a difficult one, the patient's eye may be extremely inflamed in the early postoperative period. Residual cortical material not removed during surgery may also be the cause of a severe A/C reaction (Figure 6.3). Clinically endophthalmitis tends to progress more rapidly and cause more pain than does a sterile inflammatory reaction.* A true diagnosis can sometimes be made only with an A/C or vitreous tap and culturing. Treatment consists of subconjunctival and intravitreal injection of broad-spectrum antibiotics such as vancomycin and cefazolin. Vitrectomy surgery is indicated if the media is opaque and the retina cannot be visualized.

*Postoperative inflammation or pain out of proportion to the normal postoperative findings should be considered endophthalmitis until proven otherwise.

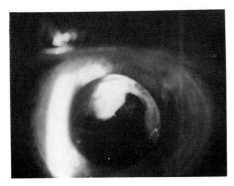

Figure 6.3
Residual cortical material, unable to be aspirated at the time of surgery, caused a severe inflammatory reaction mimicking endophthalmitis in this 64-year-old patient.

The doctor of optometry plays an important role by recognizing the signs and symptoms of endophthalmitis and notifying the surgeon immediately. Endophthalmitis is one of the few true ocular emergencies, and timely recognition and referral can save the patient's sight.

Shallow Anterior Chamber
As was mentioned previously, a shallow A/C can indicate a wound leak or pupillary block glaucoma. The surgeon should be notified if such a chamber is detected.

IRIS

Iris Atrophy
Iris atrophy can occur as a direct result of surgical trauma if:

- The surgeon attempts to remove the lens through a poorly dilated pupil.
- Surgical instruments inadvertently make contact with the iris.

Transillumination of the iris using the red reflex of the fundus is helpful in identifying areas of damage.

Traumatic Mydriasis
Sphincter damage from surgical trauma can result in a fixed, dilated pupil. This may be cosmetically troublesome to the patient and can also cause increased light sensitivity.

Pupillary Distortion
There are many reasons for pupillary distortion, or displacement secondary to cataract surgery, including:

Vitreous to the wound. Vitreous prolapse into the A/C and incarceration into the wound will drag the iris with it, creating a peaked pupil superiorly.

Iris incarceration into the wound. A wound dehiscence can result in uveal prolapse into the wound and under the conjunctiva. This can create the appearance of a sector iridectomy superiorly or in less severe cases a *watermelon-seed* shaped pupil that is displaced or peaked toward the wound.

IOLs. IOLs can cause a variety of misshaped, off-center pupils. These are discussed later in this chapter in the section entitled "Complications of IOLs."

Problems that may result from a displaced or deformed pupil aside from the undesirable cosmetic appearance include sensitivity to glare, monocular diplopia or ghost images, optical distortion from IOL positioning holes or lens edge, and reduction in visual acuity. These problems can be extremely difficult to correct. Mydriatic and miotic agents may be used diagnostically to determine if a change in pupil size will reduce symptoms. For example, a patient who notes lens-edge glare at night due to pupillary dilation may benefit from the use of a weak miotic such as ½ percent pilocarpine. If it is effective, it may then be prescribed therapeutically on an as-needed basis. Likewise, a patient with reduced acuity from a deformed, off-axis pupil might experience an improvement in vision with dilation. YAG laser coreoplasty might then be considered to permanently enlarge and recenter the pupillary aperture.

□ Late Complications

INDUCED ASTIGMATISM

Tight limbal sutures will cause corneal steepening along the axis corresponding to the location of these sutures. Since most incisions are made between 10 and 2 o'clock at the superior limbus, keratometry readings will indicate a steeper vertical meridian. This will translate into minus cylinder axis 180 (range 160 to 20). If plus cylinder is used, the axis will correspond directly to the location of the tight suture.

If with-the-rule astigmatism induced at surgery does not resolve to an acceptable level after several months, sutures will need to be cut. An *acceptable* level is typically below 1.5 diopters, or that amount of cylinder that the patient can easily adapt to and tolerate. Sutures can be cut as early as the eighth postoperative week. An almost immediate reduction in the astigmatism should be noted, but to be safe, one should wait a week or so before determining the final refraction. Suture cutting is described in Figure 6.4.

LOOSE SUTURES

Nylon sutures in postoperative cataract patients can remain intact and buried under the conjunctiva and in the cornea for many years. It is not uncommon, however, for sutures to eventually loosen, break, or become exposed (Plate 13). These patients may complain of a foreign body sensation and mucous production. The mucous is produced in response to contact between the superior tarsal plate

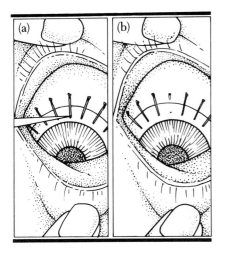

Figure 6.4
Suture cutting. Several drops of topical anesthetic are instilled into the eye. A surgical blade is used to cut the overlying conjunctiva and the involved suture(s) (a). The suture ends may retract completely into the cornea and conjunctiva. If they do not (b), one end (preferably the knotted one) should be firmly grasped with jeweler's forceps, and the entire suture removed from the eye. (Reprinted with permission of the publisher from Fingeret M, Casser L, Woodcome T. *Atlas of primary eyecare procedures.* Norwalk, Conn.: Appleton & Lange.)

and the exposed suture, resulting in a localized area of giant papillary conjunctivitis (Plate 14).*

Exposed sutures are usually easily removed using these techniques:

Loose suture (intact). A loose but intact suture must first be cut with a blade (Figure 6.5). Slide the tip of the blade under the suture, and rotate the cutting edge away from the patient. A short pulling motion should cut the suture without difficulty. There will now be two exposed ends. If one of them has a knot on it, grasp this end with jeweler's forceps and firmly pull the suture out. If there is no visible knot, pull the suture out from either end.

Loose suture (broken). If the suture is already broken and there are two exposed ends, grasp the knotted end (if it is visible) and remove it. If no knot is visible, grasp either end and pull firmly.

Exposed suture barb. An exposed suture barb can be removed with fine jeweler's forceps by firmly grasping it as close to the conjunctiva as possible (Figure 6.6). Apply steady upward pressure to completely remove the suture. Resistance may be encountered if the buried end of the suture is knotted. In this case, an effort should be made to cut the suture barb at or below the level of the conjunctiva (Figure 6.7). An exposed tip that is too small to grasp with forceps may need to be melted down with an argon laser.

---

*It is important to examine the superior bulbar conjunctiva and evert the upper lids of any postoperative patient complaining of a foreign body sensation or chronic mucoid discharge.

Figure 6.5
A loose but intact suture can cause symptoms of irritation and mucous production. The suture is grasped with forceps if necessary and then cut with a blade (a). The cut suture is grasped at the knotted end (if it is visible) with jeweler's forceps and removed (b). (Reprinted with permission of the publisher from Fingeret M, Casser L, Woodcome T. *Atlas of primary eyecare procedures.* Norwalk, Conn.: Appleton & Lange.)

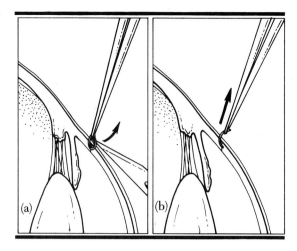

Figure 6.6
A small exposed suture barb is easily removed by grasping it with jeweler's forceps and gently pulling it out. (Reprinted with permission of the publisher from Fingeret M, Casser L, Woodcome T. *Atlas of primary eyecare procedures.* Norwalk, Conn.: Appleton & Lange.)

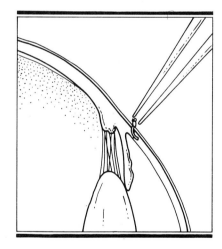

After any suture removal, a topical antibiotic should be prescribed for several days to prevent infection. Although certainly not common, cases of endophthalmitis following suture removal have been reported. Care should be taken to avoid excessive force or pulling of a knot through the conjunctiva or cornea, creating a possible entry site for bacteria into the eye.

BULLOUS KERATOPATHY

An intraocular procedure such as cataract extraction will invariably lead to some degree of endothelial cell loss. A *significant* loss of endothelial cells results in a

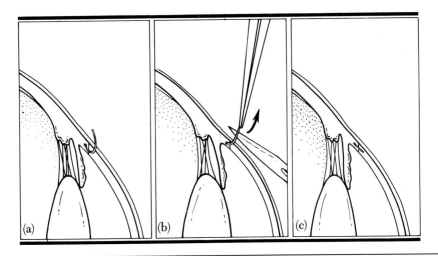

Figure 6.7   If resistance is encountered while attempting to remove a suture
barb (a), an effort should be made to cut it at its base (b) as
shown. After the suture is cut, it should retract below the
conjunctiva (c). (Reprinted with permission of the publisher
from Fingeret M, Casser L, Woodcome T. *Atlas of primary
eyecare procedures.* Norwalk, Conn.: Appleton & Lange.)

loss of integrity of the passive cell barrier, which allows fluid to enter the cornea,
and of the active endothelial pump, which allows this fluid to remain in the cornea.

A viscoelastic substance such as Healon is injected into the A/C to protect the
endothelium during surgery. While this has helped reduce corneal trauma significantly, there are patients who will eventually lose a critical number of endothelial cells and develop corneal edema. Other factors that contribute to
endothelial cell loss and corneal edema are:

- Preexisting guttata or Fuch's dystrophy
- Trauma from insertion of the IOL or endothelial touch from dislocated IOL
- Vitreous loss with intact anterior hyaloid face contacting the endothelium.

Corneal decompensation is defined as loss of endothelial integrity leading to
intake of fluid. Clinically this process involves fluid accumulation in the stroma,
presenting initially as fine vertical stria and progressing to stromal folds, thick-
ening, and opacification (Figure 6.8). The fluid eventually affects the corneal
epithelium as well by causing the formation of microcysts. These microcysts may
eventually coalesce into bullae, referred to as aphakic bullous keratopathy (ABK)
or pseudophakic bullous keratopathy (PBK) (Figure 6.9). The bullae may eventually rupture, causing significant pain.

Stromal or epithelial edema typically produces symptoms of gradual VA loss
with onset several months to years after surgery. VA is often poor on awakening
in the morning but clears somewhat as the day progresses. This is related to

Figure 6.8
Stromal folds seen in the early postoperative period usually resolve completely. When seen several months to years after surgery, they often signal corneal decompensation.

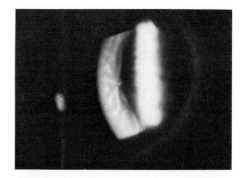

Figure 6.9
Intake of fluid into the cornea eventually results in epithelial edema, seen clinically as microcysts (a), which coalesce into bullae (b) that can eventually break (c) causing significant pain.

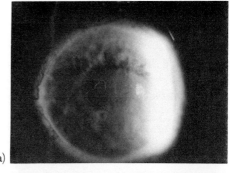

(a)

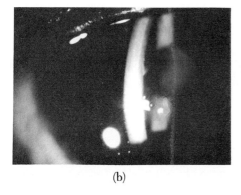

(b)

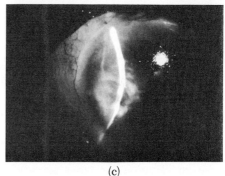

(c)

increased edema with lid closure during sleep and relative dehydration as the eyes are open during the day. Patients may also complain of tearing, light sensitivity, foreign body sensation, and at times significant pain.

Management of corneal decompensation includes:

- *Hypertonic saline drops or ointment.* Some common brands include Muro 128 (2 or 5 percent) solution or Muro 128 (5 percent) ointment, both preservative free, or Adsorbonac (2 or 5 percent) solution. All are available without a prescription. The initial dosage will depend on the patient's symptoms and on biomicroscopic findings. Examples of possible treatment regimens are listed in

Slit Lamp Finding	Treatment	Initial Dosage
Early stromal edema Fine striae	2% or 5% hypertonic saline drops	QID
Moderate stromal edema Early folds Early microcysts	5% drops (5% hypertonic saline ointment added later if needed)	Q 3–4h QHS
Advanced stromal edema Large folds Bullae formation	5% drops 5% ointment Hairdryer Possible corneal transplant	Q 1–2h QHS

Table 6.4   Suggested Use of Hypertonic Saline for Bullous Keratopathy

Table 6.4. For those patients who note improvement in VA or comfort, emphasis should be placed on the need for long-term use.

• *Portable hairdryer* (on a medium heat setting and held at arm's length) blown into the eyes when symptomatic.

• *Bandage contact lens* (disposable lens or collagen shield) in cases of severe discomfort or broken bullae

• *Corneal transplant surgery*

Hypertonic saline and the hairdryer are short-term solutions to a problem that in many cases will require surgical correction with corneal transplantation (penetrating keratoplasty). ABK and PBK are the most common indications for penetrating keratoplasty in the United States. If the IOL is responsible for the corneal decompensation, it may have to be removed or exchanged at the same time the transplant is performed.

EPITHELIAL DOWNGROWTH

The growth of epithelial cells into the A/C is a catastrophic but fortunately very rare complication of cataract surgery. It can occur with other intraocular surgery as well but is most commonly seen following cataract extraction. It is assumed to be caused by a poorly closed wound with corneal or conjunctival epithelial cells growing down into the A/C. A sheet of epithelium can eventually cover the endothelium, iris, and trabecular meshwork and lead to glaucoma, corneal decompensation, and permanent acuity loss. Many surgical techniques have been used to treat this condition, including corneal transplantation, removal of involved iris, and cryotherapy. None has met with a high degree of success.

REBOUND IRITIS

Weeks or months after the normal postoperative inflammatory reaction has disappeared patients will occasionally present with the acute onset of a red, light

Figure 6.10
Capsular fibrosis (courtesy of
American Academy of
Ophthalmology).

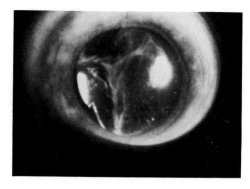

sensitive eye. If cell and flare is noted in the A/C, the patient probably has a rebound iritis. This iritis has no apparent underlying etiology and responds extremely well to topical steroids. The dosage (depending on the amount of cell and flare) usually ranges from q.2h to q.4h. Once improvement is noted, the steroids should be tapered *very slowly* over several weeks in order to avoid another rebound episode.

POSTERIOR CAPSULAR OPACIFICATION

Posterior capsular opacification (PCO) is one of the most common *late* complications of extracapsular cataract surgery. Also referred to as a *secondary cataract* or *after-cataract,* this problem is usually noticed by patients several months to years after the original surgery. The rate of occurrence and time of onset in part depend on how meticulously the surgeon polishes the posterior capsule, but opacification will eventually occur in a large percentage of patients undergoing extracapsular cataract extraction (ECCE) despite careful efforts to prevent it. Patient symptoms include gradual VA loss in the operated eye, occasionally accompanied by glare or monocular ghost images.

Clinically PCO can present in one of two ways:

1. *Capsular fibrosis.* The posterior capsule wrinkles and opacifies, forming thickened whitish bands (Figure 6.10).

2. *Pearl formation.* Lens epithelial cells enlarge and proliferate, forming *Elschnig's pearls.* As these pearls spread, opacification of the capsule occurs (Figure 6.11).

The posterior capsule should be evaluated for opacification both pre- and postdilation using the biomicroscope. Before dilation, observe the location of the pupil in relation to the area of capsular opacification. After dilation, evaluate the entire capsule using both direct illumination and retroillumination.

Using the Hruby or 90 diopter lens, the next step is to determine the view of the fundus *through* the opacified capsule. As with a cataract, the view *in* should correspond to the patient's view *out* (VA) if the capsule is responsible for the acuity loss. The potential acuity meter, useful in predicting postoperative acuity

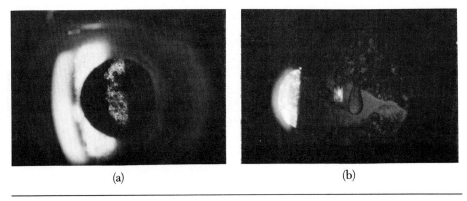

(a)   (b)

Figure 6.11   Elschnig pearls of the posterior capsule as seen in direct illumination (a) and retroillumination in a different patient (b).

prior to cataract surgery, does not typically provide meaningful information when performed through a cloudy capsule.

Treatment

Capsular opacification was once treated by creating a surgical opening or *discission* in the clouded capsule. The Neodymium: YAG (yttrium aluminum garnet) laser developed in the late 1970s has rendered surgical techniques obsolete. Using infrared wavelengths of 1060 nanometers of light, the YAG laser relies on a principle known as *optical breakdown*. Molecular bonds are broken by a shock wave or microexplosion created by a short, single burst of highly focused laser energy. This shock wave cuts or opens the target tissue, creating an audible snap. Although the YAG laser is used primarily to perform capsulotomies, other uses in managing postoperative complications include:

- Iridotomies in pupillary block glaucoma
- Lysis of vitreous bands to the cataract wound
- Coreoplasty or reshaping the pupillary aperture to improve VA
- Synechialysis, which breaks iris adhesions to the anterior lens capsule or IOL surface

A YAG capsulotomy is a fast, simple, in-office procedure requiring only topical anesthesia. It can be performed with or without a special laser contact lens (Figure 6.12), which stabilizes the eye and lids and allows more efficient delivery of laser energy. Once the patient is positioned in the instrument, an initial energy setting is selected. YAG energy is rated in millijoules with an initial setting of .7 to 1.0 millijoules. The energy is gradually increased if necessary until the capsular tissue is disrupted (Figure 6.13). Patients should experience a fairly rapid and often dramatic improvement in acuity. Although uncommon, possible complications to watch for following YAG capsulotomy include:

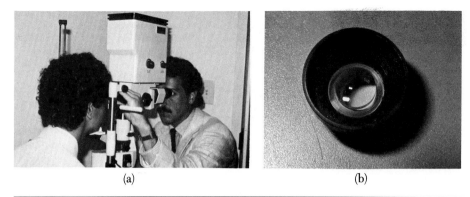

(a)   (b)

Figure 6.12   The YAG laser is a relatively compact instrument (a), ideal for in-office use. A special contact lens (b) can be used to stabilize the eye and enhance laser delivery.

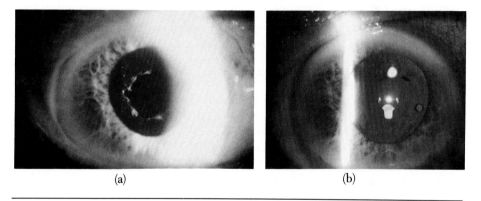

(a)   (b)

Figure 6.13   A completed YAG capsulotomy as seen in direct illumination (a) and retroillumination (b). (Courtesy of Cliff Courtenay, O.D.)

Intraocular pressure spikes. Patients can develop very high spikes in intraocular pressure soon after the YAG is performed. For this reason, some surgeons pretreat with the pressure-lowering medication Iopidine (apraclonidine) prior to the YAG procedure. It is good clinical protocol to keep patients in the office for a pressure check one hour after the capsulotomy. Should elevated pressure be noted, treatment with a topical beta blocker is usually very effective.

Iritis. A small amount of cell and flare in the A/C is not unusual following a YAG procedure. Some surgeons will routinely put these patients on a topical steroid. Others reserve the use of steroids for those patients exhibiting an unusual amount of inflammation. Capsular debris seen floating in the A/C may be mistaken for cell and flare.

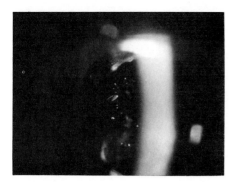

Figure 6.14
A large nick surrounded by several smaller pits results from improper focusing of the YAG laser beam.

Capsular opening too small. Following the laser procedure, the VA should improve. If it does not, look at the size of the opening to be sure it is adequate (Figure 6.13). If it is, consider the possibility of either a preexisting fundus abnormality or a retinal complication related to the YAG laser procedure itself.

Cystoid macular edema (CME). This should be suspected in a patient whose VA improves following YAG capsulotomy and then decreases gradually over the next few weeks or months. The exact incidence of CME following a secondary YAG capsulotomy is unknown, but probably ranges between 2 percent and 4 percent. The etiology is unknown, but some proposed mechanisms are listed in the section on retinal complications below.

Retinal detachment (RD). One of the most serious complications following YAG capsulotomy is a retinal detachment. Any break in the posterior capsule, performed either surgically during cataract extraction or with the laser after surgery, increases the risk of RD. The incidence of RD following YAG capsulotomy is very low, but if it occurs it will usually do so within the first 6 months to a year after the procedure. Patients who have undergone YAG capsulotomy should have a dilated fundus examination within three months after the procedure or sooner if they note symptoms of flashes, floaters, or vision or field loss.

Pitted IOL. Pitting or nicking of the IOL can occur if the YAG laser is aimed improperly (Figure 6.14). Pit marks are usually of no consequence, but if enough are present, the patient may note glare or a slight reduction in vision.

RETINA

Cystoid Macular Edema

Cystoid macular edema (CME) is a well-documented complication of cataract surgery and posterior capsulotomy. There is a high incidence of CME with intracapsular techniques, especially when vitreous is incarcerated in the wound. This is known as the *Irvine-Gass syndrome*. The incidence of CME in intracapsular surgery varies depending on the study read. A distinction should be made between CME with vision loss (incidence 2–10 percent) and CME without visual symptoms but demonstrable by fluorescein angiography (incidence 40–60 percent). It is well known that the incidence of CME is significantly lower with extracapsular tech-

Figure 6.15
The characteristic fluorescein angiography appearance of CME as shown in the late stage of the study.

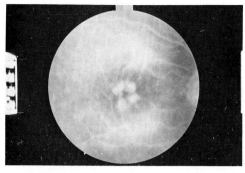

niques. In the hands of an experienced extracapsular surgeon, clinically significant CME is an infrequent complication.

CME is characterized by gradual, progressive acuity loss in the operated eye several months to years after the procedure. VA can range anywhere from 20/20 to 20/200 but is usually in the 20/50 to 20/80 range.

Clinically, there are several manifestations of the disease. Using fundus biomicroscopy at a high magnification setting (typically 25x), a yellowish nodule or dot will be observed under the fovea along with a noticeably absent light reflex. As more fluid collects, a "honeycomb" appearance becomes evident, with small cystic cavities extending out from the central foveal area (Plate 15). The definitive diagnosis is made with fluorescein angiography, with its characteristic early leakage and late staining petaloid pattern (Figure 6.15).

CME is not only associated with surgery but can also be a complication of other disease entities including diabetic retinopathy, posterior uveitis/vitritis, retinal vein occlusions, and exudative macular degeneration. There are many theories regarding the pathogenesis of CME, including inflammation, mechanical traction and prostaglandin production. Recent treatment strategies have been directed at inhibiting prostaglandin synthesis and inflammation, using:

- Oral or topical nonsteroidal anti-inflammatory drugs (NSAIDs) such as oral Indocin (indomethacin) or topical Ocufen (flurbiprofen)
- Oral or topical steroids
- Subconjunctival or periocular steroid injections
- Oral carbonic anhydrase inhibitors
- Surgical management including IOL exchange with anterior vitrectomy or YAG vitreolysis to relieve traction of incarcerated vitreous to the wound

Because of a lack of controlled studies, it is uncertain which if any of these treatment strategies is most effective. Many cases will resolve on their own, especially if VA is better than 20/50. If the edema does not resolve, a lamellar or full thickness macular hole could result. This may lead to permanent central acuity loss, often 20/200 or less. If the patient is symptomatic, some form of therapy should probably be instituted.

Retinal Detachment

Probably the most serious and permanently debilitating complication following cataract surgery is retinal detachment (RD) (Plate 16). Most RDs occur within the first three years following surgery. Prompt recognition of the problem by the patient and doctor will improve the chance for surgical and functional success, although once the macula is detached it is unlikely that vision will be completely restored.

The incidence of RD, like that of CME, is much higher in intracapsular surgery than it is when extracapsular techniques are used. This is most likely related to the loss of the capsular barrier and anterior shifting of vitreous with resultant vitreoretinal traction. While flashes, floaters, and vision loss will often signal a problem, some patients will present with asymptomatic tears or detachments. These changes are often extremely peripheral and easily overlooked, necessitating full dilation and careful indirect ophthalmoscopy of all aphakes and pseudophakes on a routine basis. Scleral indentation may be useful if the view of the peripheral retina is obscured by capsular haze or the IOL. Timely referral to a qualified vitreoretinal specialist is extremely important.

___ ■_____

COMPLICATIONS OF INTRAOCULAR LENSES

Contemporary cataract surgery techniques involve the implantation of an IOL. There have been tremendous advances in lens design since the early 1970s when lens implantation began. Early lenses such as the iris-plane and iris-fixated designs were associated with a number of serious complications and are no longer used. These gave way to A/C and posterior chamber IOLs, which are used successfully on many patients today. Regardless of the type of IOL used, however, complications related specifically to the lens implant do occur.

☐ Incorrect Power

One objective of successful implant surgery is to leave the patient with the desired refractive correction. The usual goal is to render the eye emmetropic, but the surgeon should be advised if a specific correction is needed. For example, a patient who has already undergone implant surgery in one eye ends up with a final refraction of -3.00 sphere. A decision must be made either to match this refraction in the fellow eye or to try for emmetropia and create a monovision system.

The appropriate IOL power for a given eye is determined by entering keratometry readings, axial length measurements, and the desired postoperative re-

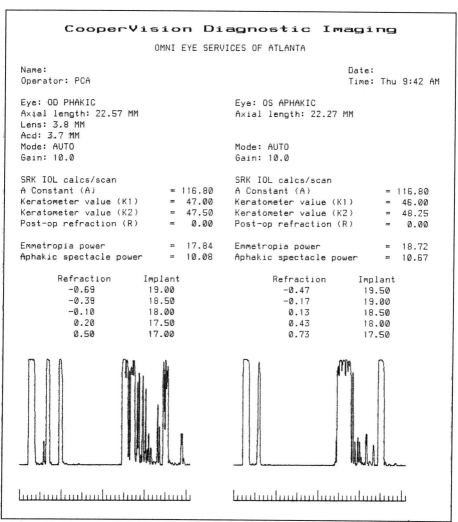

Figure 6.16   An A-scan axial length reading with IOL power calculations.

fraction into one of several formulas built into the software of the A-scan instrument. The instrument then calculates the appropriate lens power with ranges on the plus and minus side (Figure 6.16). It is important to realize how critical these measurements can be:

1mm error in axial length = 2.5 diopter change in IOL power

1 diopter change in keratometry reading = .9 diopter change in IOL power

Fortunately most IOL calculations are performed by competent doctors or technicians. Delegating these tests (A-scan and K readings) to an untrained staff member, however, can have significant consequences. The *7-diopter surprise* indicates a final refraction that is very different from the intended result. These patients are difficult to manage refractively and may need to be fit with contact lenses to correct the anisometropia. In some cases, the surgeon is forced to remove the IOL and replace it with one of the correct power.

Some warning signs of incorrect keratometry or A-scan readings include:

- Axial length measurements outside normal range (22 to 25mm)
- Keratometry readings outside normal range (40 to 46 diopters)
- Large difference in measurements between eyes:

> axial length: >0.3mm difference
> keratometry: >1.0 diopter difference in either meridian

□ Malposition

Another important objective of IOL surgery is to position the lens in the eye so that proper centration is maintained. A significantly decentered lens can cause a variety of problems, including reduced vision, glare, and structural damage to the eye. Decentration or dislocation of IOLs was seen much more commonly in the early iris-fixated lenses than it is today. Any type of IOL can become malpositioned, however.

Iris-fixated lenses. If patients with this lens are mistakenly dilated, the lens can end up on the retina or in the A/C (Figure 6.17). These lenses have caused a great deal of damage to the cornea due to partial or total anterior dislocation and endothelial touch.*

A/C lenses. Historically rigid A/C lenses represented a significant improvement over iris-fixated lenses because they were less likely to decenter. This could still occur, however, if the lens was undersized. The newer A/C lenses with flexible haptics, used commonly in secondary implant procedures, are not prone to decentration or subluxation. The pupils of these patients can be fully dilated.

Posterior chamber lenses. The lens of choice in extracapsular cataract surgery is the posterior chamber lens (PC IOL). This lens design has solved many problems created by its predecessors, resulting in increased stability. Refinements in surgical technique such as capsulorhexis and in-the-bag fixation along with improvements in lens design have helped minimize PC IOL displacement.

Caution: This is the only IOL seen clinically that contraindicates routine dilation. If dilation is essential, judicious use of a mild mydriatic such as 0.5 percent tropicamide is in order. The pupil should be closely observed, and pilocarpine should be kept readily available to reverse dilation if necessary. Many of these lenses become permanently adherent to the iris, making dilation difficult even if one were to attempt it.

Figure 6.17
A Binkhorst four-loop iris-fixated
lens in the anterior chamber after
inadvertent dilation.

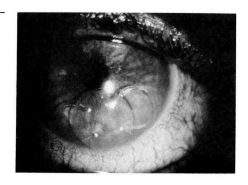

The lens, however, is still prone to decentration in a small percentage of cases. Malposition of a PC IOL can occur in one of three ways:

1. *Pupil capture.* This occurs when some portion of the IOL optic is caught in the pupil and becomes lodged anterior to the iris. There is a chance it can be repositioned pharmacologically if it is detected early. Unfortunately pupil capture may occur without any symptoms. By the time the patient is seen, permanent synechiae have formed. If the pupil is decentered significantly, VA may be reduced (Figure 6.18).

2. *Decentration.* Slight shifting of a PC IOL from the centered position is common and causes no visual symptoms. If the lens becomes significantly decentered, however, the patient may experience reduced vision, glare, monocular ghost images, or arcs of light. Capsular bag fixation and the integrity of the zonules are extremely important for lens stability. If the inferior capsule ruptures, the inferior zonules are damaged, or the haptic is not in the bag, the lens can drop inferiorly. This is known as the *sunset syndrome* (Figure 6.19). Less commonly seen is the *sunrise syndrome,* caused by damage to the superior zonules. The lens can also shift nasally or temporally.

3. *Windshield wiper syndrome.* An undersized PC IOL may move during head and eye movements, causing fluctuating vision and possibly chronic uveitis. This rare complication requires either suturing of the lens to the iris or replacement with a lens of the proper size.

Figure 6.18
Pupil capture can result in
synechiae of the iris to the IOL, an
eccentric pupil, and resultant
acuity loss.

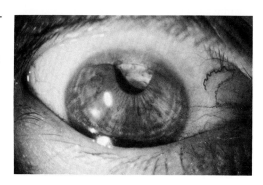

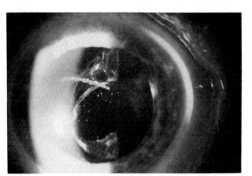

Figure 6.19
Sunset syndrome. The PC IOL is seen displaced inferiorly, causing the patient to notice lens edge glare and visual distortion.

☐ Inflammation

Ideally an IOL should be implanted in such a way as to avoid contact with the iris and vascular uveal tissue. If it is not, chronic intraocular inflammation can result. The old, poorly designed, iris-fixated and A/C lenses caused mechanical irritation of the iris and angle with resultant chronic iritis. A variation of this has been termed the UGH (uveitis-glaucoma-hyphema) syndrome. The constant contact of the implant with the iris and trabecular meshwork caused uveitis as well as recurrent hyphemas and secondary glaucoma. Although it has been reported with the newer A/C and PC IOL, it is rarely seen clinically anymore.

Any type of chronic uveitis can cause inflammatory precipitates on the IOL surface. These precipitates, similar in appearance to keratic precipitates on the corneal endothelium, can often be eliminated with aggressive topical steroid therapy. If the inflammation is not responsive to therapy, one must consider an entity known as *toxic lens syndrome*. While the etiology is not known, this syndrome probably represents an immune response to the lens material or to defective components of the lens. The only effective therapy for this rare complication is removal of the implant. The toxic lens syndrome and its accompanying sterile uveitis must be distinguished from true infectious endophthalmitis.

☐ Infection

An IOL implant may be the means by which bacteria enter the eye during surgery, leading to endophthalmitis. The signs and symptoms are the same as have been previously described, regardless of the etiology.

One exception is a low-grade, smoldering inflammatory reaction that can begin weeks or months after surgery that is caused by the organism Propionibacterium acnes. This anerobic, gram-positive organism is found in the normal flora of the eye. It was previously thought to be nonpathogenic but has been identified in the posterior capsular bag (between the capsule and IOL) as a cause of chronic endophthalmitis. In some cases, a white plaque is seen peripherally between the posterior capsule and the implant. Often the only effective treatment for this type of endophthalmitis is removal of the IOL and the posterior capsule.

Figure 6.20
The Copeland iris plane lens causing a square pupil. Two of the haptics are in front of the iris and two are behind the iris at one and seven o'clock.

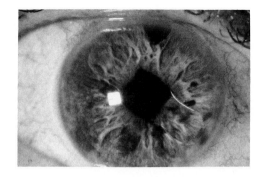

Figure 6.21
The Choyce A/C lens, no longer used, created a vertically oval pupil.

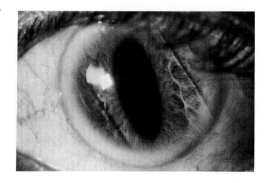

□ Corneal Trauma

Bullous keratopathy can be related specifically to the endothelial trauma induced by the IOL during implantation or subsequently by intermittent endothelial touch. PBK was more commonly seen when iris-fixated and A/C lenses were in widespread use. Most patients who developed PBK from these lenses in the late 1970s have either had corneal transplant surgery or are no longer living.

Patients undergoing ECCE with a posterior chamber implant can develop PBK, but the risk is significantly lower. The cautious surgeon will carefully evaluate the endothelium preoperatively, and in a suspect cornea will use viscoelastic substances and avoid phacoemulsification to prevent any unnecessary cell loss and resultant corneal decompensation.

□ Iris Trauma

There are a number of ways the iris can be traumatized by an IOL, including:

Pupil distortion. Iris-fixated and iris plane lenses became well known for creating distorted pupils. The Copeland iris plane lens commonly caused a square pupil (Figure 6.20) and permanent synechiae to the IOL. The early A/C lenses

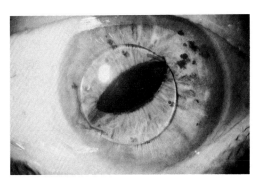

Figure 6.22
A PC IOL that was displaced into the anterior chamber, creating pupillary distortion. The vision was unaffected.

caused oval or cat's eye pupils as can be seen in Figure 6.21. PC IOLs can occasionally become displaced into the A/C, causing a distorted pupil (Figure 6.22).

Iris atrophy. Iris-fixated lenses can cause iris atrophy. A/C lenses can actually erode through the iris, allowing the opposite footplate to rotate anteriorly and contact the corneal endothelium.

Iris tuck. Iris tuck occurs when the haptic or footplate of the anterior chamber IOL is imbedded in peripheral iris tissue, causing a distorted pupil.

*Postoperative inflammation or pain out of proportion to the normal postoperative findings should be considered endophthalmitis until proven otherwise.

*It is important to examine the superior bulbar conjunctiva and evert the upper lids of any postoperative patient complaining of a foreign body sensation or chronic mucoid discharge.

7

Co-management, Medicolegal, and Reimbursement Considerations

□

Co-management of cataract patients between the doctor of optometry and the ophthalmic surgeon has become such an integral part of the health care system that it is recognized by the Health Care Financing Administration (HCFA), the governmental organization that oversees the Medicare system. The American Academy of Ophthalmology's Code of Ethics also recognizes this relationship, stating that:

> Ethical Rules 7 (Delegation of Services) and 8 (Postoperative Care) would not preclude an Academy member from referring patients to a non-ophthalmological physician . . . for those aspects of postoperative care that are not within the unique competence of the ophthalmologist . . . provided that the person is legally entitled and professionally trained, experienced, and qualified to provide the particular services.*

This relationship places increased responsibility on the optometrist in the areas of communication with the surgeon, documentation, and standards of care. These medicolegal issues will be discussed, along with reimbursement considerations.

■

HISTORY OF CO-MANAGEMENT

Co-management was an idea conceived and developed in the early 1980s. Doctors of optometry were frustrated with the up-to-then traditional model of eye care, which involved one-way medical and surgical referrals to ophthalmologists. There was little, if any, correspondence from the surgeon to the referring optometrist.

*Argus, March 1992, p. 6.

Patients and their families were often discouraged from returning to their primary care doctor of optometry. Postoperative cataract patients were either sent back long after the surgery was performed for a prescription change, or not sent back at all. An insightful group of doctors in Georgia established the first true optometric consultation/co-management center based on the following principles:

- Patients sent to a surgeon by an optometrist should be sent back to that optometrist after surgical treatment is completed.
- Doctors of optometry can and should play an active role in the postoperative care of *their* patients.
- The co-management center should serve as an extension of the optometrist's practice by providing consultative and educational support.
- The center should be affiliated with highly trained surgeons and state-of-the-art equipment and diagnostic services.

This model of care has been recognized and imitated by leading ophthalmic surgeons nationwide. Co-management of the cataract patient has been very successful because of:

Better geographic distribution of optometrists. Care is accessible to patients who otherwise might have to travel some distance. A patient may still have to travel to get to the best surgeon, but many of the follow-up visits can be done closer to home. With easier access to care, patients are more likely to keep their follow-up appointments.

Increased communication. The doctor of optometry knows the surgeon's postoperative protocol and has been trained to handle minor complications. The optometrist also knows when to send the patient back in the unlikely event of a major complication.

Cost containment. The surgery and postoperative care are delivered by both providers at no additional cost to patients or third party carriers. *Ongoing* care can also be provided closer to home at a typically lower fee.

Peer review. The referring optometrist evaluates each surgical case and quickly becomes familiar with the surgeon's results. Should the results be consistently poor, the optometrist will seek these services elsewhere. Since the patient and other medical specialists are generally unable to evaluate the skills of a cataract surgeon, this peer review selection process enhances the quality of care delivered.

The Batelle study (Rivicki, 1989) revealed that 86 percent of all co-managed cases evaluated had final visual acuity (VA) of 20/40 or better. The complication rate was equivalent to, or lower than, that seen in patients managed by the surgeon only. The study, which retrospectively evaluated data from five major co-management centers around the country, revealed that co-managed care is extremely beneficial to the patient if:

- The surgeon is well qualified.
- The optometrist is well trained in examining the postoperative eye.
- Good communication between the two professionals exists.
- There is a clear understanding of postoperative protocol.
- There is a coordinated effort to ensure compliance with follow-up visits.

The study found that "optometrists can and do provide quality patient care following cataract surgery, and that patient outcomes are comparable regardless of whether postoperative care is delivered by optometrists and ophthalmic surgeons, or by ophthalmic surgeons alone."

■

MEDICOLEGAL ASPECTS OF CATARACT CARE

□ Standard of Care

Eye care practitioners are held to a *standard of care* that becomes more specifically defined as time goes on. Standard of care is a term used a great deal in conjunction with medical malpractice cases. If doctors adhere to the standard of care, and their actions do not cause patients harm, malpractice has not occurred. Exactly what is the standard of care when performing a routine examination or evaluating a particular ocular disorder, and who sets the standard? Traditionally state boards of optometry set standards for their peers. Courts are now determining standards, however, based on the outcome of malpractice cases. Doctors of optometry in many instances are being held to the same standards of care as are doctors of medicine.

In order to protect both optometrist and patient, a certain battery of basic tests should be performed on all new patients, including cataract patients. These tests were reviewed in Chapter 2. If this basic testing leads one to suspect other problems such as glaucoma, neurological disease, or retinal abnormalities, additional testing can be performed or ordered, for example:

- Formal automated visual fields
- Gonioscopy
- Color vision
- Amsler grid testing

- Radiologic studies (computerized tomography [CT] and/or magnetic resonance imaging [MRI])
- Blood chemistry
- Carotid doppler ultrasound studies

If the appropriate testing is performed on every patient in a systematic, consistent manner, nothing will be left to chance. Once a cataract is detected, do not assume that it is the only reason for the vision loss. Be alert for more insidious disorders coexisting with the cataracts such as low tension glaucoma or peripheral retinal disease. Maintaining a minimum standard of care will benefit patient and practitioner alike.

☐ Recordkeeping/Documentation

A good way to force oneself to perform a basic battery of tests on each patient is to design an examination form with a place to record each test (Figure 7.1). If a test is inadvertently omitted, the blank space will serve as a reminder that it needs to be done.

Recording test results properly is as important as doing the test itself. Document all findings thoroughly, and record them completely and legibly. The more detailed the record, the safer the practitioner will be. Compare the following two records:

Record 1:   Anterior segment—clear

Record 2:   Lids, lashes—clear
Conjunctiva—quiet
Cornea—endothelial pigment
A/C—deep, quiet
Iris—clear
Lens—early nuclear yellowing

Record 2 is obviously much more defensible in the event of a malpractice suit. A complete record is a positive reflection of a doctor's clinical competence.

Never go back and add, delete, or change anything on an already established exam form. If you need to add information obtained on a different date, record it as a separate entry. Always sign your charts, and if others (such as technicians or interns) are writing in the chart, have them sign it as well.

Another excellent form of documentation is photography. Anterior segment photography or videophotography allows the practitioner to record lenticular opacities or postoperative complications. More important is the ability to document a fundus lesion or disc anomaly that might affect postoperative acuity. Fundus photography also enhances one's ability to follow the progress of retinal disease or glaucoma over time.

EXAMINATION:

Visual Acuity: (with/without Rx)

RE: ph   Near

LE: ph   Near

Present Glasses:

RE:

LE:

Auto-Refraction and VA:

RE:

LE:

Refraction and VA: Lights On

RE:

LE:

Confrontation Fields:

LE   RE

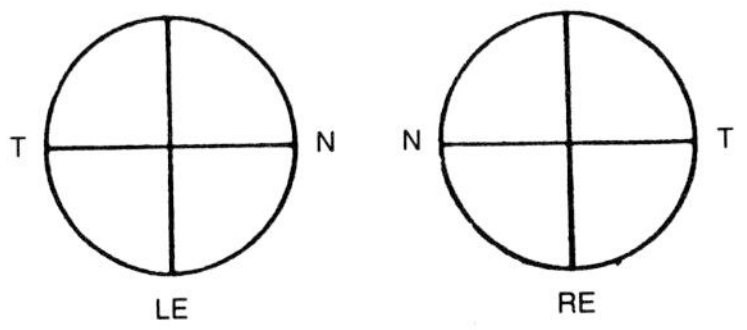

PAM: Glare Test:

RE: RE:

LE: LE:

Visual Function Tests: Blood Pressure

(Amsler Grid, color, BFE)

RE:

LE:

Motility:

Pupils: RE:

          LE:

External: K RE:

                LE:

Slit Lamp   RE   LE

Lids & lashes

Conjunctiva

Cornea

A.C.

Iris

Lens

Tension (Applanation)   Time of measurement:

RE:

LE: Last medications:

Figure 7.1   An example of a new patient examination form with areas provided to record each test.

☐ Referral versus Consultation

Technically speaking, there is a difference between referral and consultation. A true referral involves turning the patient over completely to another medical practitioner with no responsibility for the patient during the treatment period. Consultation, on the other hand, implies co-management; for example, sending a patient for surgery but taking responsibility for postoperative care immediately after the surgery. According to Classé (1989), this joint undertaking results in significantly more responsibility and liability should a problem occur. Both parties, not just the surgeon, can be sued in the event of a complication. This underscores the importance of carefully selecting and recommending highly qualified surgeons or other medical specialists. While it may be less convenient to send patients a longer distance to a more qualified specialist, it may be in the best interest of all concerned.

☐ Tracking Follow-up Visits

Once the doctor of optometry enters into a co-management relationship with a surgeon, the responsibility increases dramatically. It is critical that postoperative follow-up appointments be kept. If they are not, a system should be in place to document the missed visit and reschedule it. Computers can assist in this task although many offices still rely on manual techniques (Figure 7.2). If patients cannot be contacted, a *registered letter* should be sent asking them to call the office to reschedule. Keep an accurate record of phone calls made and letters sent.

If postoperative cataract patients develop complications, they may need to be

---

NO SHOW

DATE APPT MISSED _____

_____ Left Message	_____ Phone Disconnected
_____ Will Call Back To Reschedule	_____ Phone # Unpublished
_____ Out Of Town	_____ Sick
_____ Does Not Wish To Reschedule	_____ Sent Letter
_____ Unable to Contact	_____ Appt. Resc.

Figure 7.2 By documenting the status of each *no-show* patient, rescheduling will not be left to chance.

sent back to the surgeon. If so, *be sure to make the appointment for the patient in a timely manner.* Record the appointment time and date on the examination form and on a card that patients can take with them. If they will not allow you to make the appointment, document this in the record and give them the referral information in writing.

□ Communication with the Surgeon

Co-managing doctors of optometry should take time to inform surgeons of the results of each postoperative examination. Just as optometrists have come to expect detailed reports from secondary and tertiary care specialists, so should they assume the responsibility of communicating with the surgeons on each cataract patient's progress. This is often done informally by phone but should probably be documented using some type of reporting form that may also serve as the postoperative examination form (Figure 7.3).

■ REIMBURSEMENT

While the main goal of each practitioner should always be to provide the highest level of care possible to all patients, it is important to be reimbursed appropriately for that care. To this end, a thorough understanding of the insurance system, including Medicare, Medicaid, health maintenance organizations (HMOs), and private carriers, is mandatory.

In order to describe to insurance carriers what procedures have been done and why, it is important to be completely familiar with CPT (current procedural terminology) codes, ICD-9 (international classification of disease) codes, and local *carrier-assigned* codes. CPT codes are procedure codes used to describe to the carrier *which* tests were performed. Those related to the pre- and postoperative cataract evaluation are listed in Tables 7.1 through 7.3. ICD-9 codes are diagnosis codes used to explain *why* these tests were performed. Those codes applicable to cataract patients are listed in Table 7.4.

Once a diagnosis of cataract is made, Medicare and private carriers will allow coverage for a complete eye examination, such as a 92004 (initial exam—comprehensive). The potential acuity meter (PAM), glare testing, and brightness acuity testing (BAT) are considered to be minor diagnostic tests that are included in the eye examination, and therefore will not be covered by Medicare.* Other ancillary tests such as visual fields or photography will be covered. A-scan ultrasonography to measure axial length of the eye will be reimbursed only in conjunction with

*Some private insurance companies may cover one or more of these tests.

```
┌─────────────────────────────────────────────────────────────────────┐
│                        POST-OP REPORT FORM                            │
│                                                                       │
│   PATIENT'S NAME: _____  DATE:_____  │
│                                                                       │
│   DOCTOR:_____   │
│                                                                       │
│   CATARACT EXTRACTION  O_____   _____    │
│                          Eye              Surgery Date                │
│                                                                       │
│   CC: _____    │
│                                                                       │
│   MEDICATIONS:   _____  O_____   QID  TID  BID  QD _____      │
│                                  Eye     (CIRCLE ONE)                  │
│                                                                       │
│                  _____  O_____   QID  TID  BID  QD _____      │
│                                  Eye     (CIRCLE ONE)                  │
│                                                                       │
│   ANY ADDITIONAL DROPS: _____     │
└─────────────────────────────────────────────────────────────────────┘
```

*** EXAMINATION OF OPERATED EYE ***

POST-OP VISIT (CIRCLE ONE)   WEEK   1 2 3 4 5 6 7 8 9 10 11 12 Other_____

VA WITHOUT CORRECTION 20/_____   PINHOLE 20/_____

REFRACTION _____VA_____ KERATOMETRY _____

SLIT LAMP EXAM   (CIRCLE WITH COMMENTS)   CONFRONTATION
                                                VISUAL FIELDS_____

   WOUND   INTACT _____   SEPARATION _____

   CORNEA   CLEAR _____ STRIAE _____ EDEMA _____

   ANTERIOR CHAMBER   0   1+   2+   3+   4+   CELL/FLARE

   IOL STATUS   CENTERED _____ DECENTERED _____

   POST. CAPSULE CLEAR _____ HAZY _____ WRINKLED _____

   MACULA   NORMAL _____ CYSTOID EDEMA _____ AMD _____

TENSIONS (APPLANATION)   _____mm Hg at _____a.m./p.m.

   FUNDUS   _____

IMPRESSON AND PLAN:_____

                       _____

                       _____

Signature: _____

**If any severe pain and/or decrease in vision develops,
an immediate consultation is indicated.**

FOLD TOP COPY AND SEND TO OMNI • SECOND COPY REFERRING DOCTORS' RECORD

Figure 7.3   An example of a postoperative reporting form. One copy goes to
the surgeon and another stays in the patient's file, doubling as
an examination form.

Procedure	CPT Code
Initial examination—comprehensive	92004
Established patient—comprehensive	92014
Visual field examination:	
Intermediate (screening suprathreshold)	92082
Extended (threshold)	92083
Fundus photography	92250
External ocular photography (slit lamp)	92285
Specular endothelial microscopy	92286
Electroretinography (ERG)	92275
Visual evoked potential (VEP)	92280
Potential acuity meter (PAM)*	Local carrier assigned code: W0001–Z9999
Glare testing/contrast sensitivity/BAT*	92284

*For Medicare patients, these tests are considered part of the eye examination codes and thus cannot be billed separately.

Table 7.1   CPT Codes Used in the Preoperative Cataract Evaluation

Procedure	CPT Code
ECCE—no IOL	66940
ECCE—with IOL	66984
Intracapsular cataract extraction (ICCE) with IOL	66983
Secondary IOL implantation	66985
YAG laser capsulotomy	66821

Table 7.2   CPT Codes Used in Cataract Surgery and Related Procedures

cataract surgery. B-scan ultrasonography will also be covered if a mature cataract is present and a retinal detachment or tumor is suspected. Endothelial cell photography is covered when patients meet one or more of the criteria: the presence of a corneal dystrophy, edema, or guttata; a history of previous intraocular surgery; or a planned phacoemulsification or a secondary implant procedure.

The filing of the *preoperative* evaluation is the same regardless of whether the patient is covered by Medicare, Medicaid, or private insurance. There are significant differences in coding, however, as concerns the *postoperative* follow-up care.

Service	CPT Code
Postoperative visits within 90 days of surgery	
Routine or urgent visits related to surgery—file all visits as one	Modifier 55 preceded by surgical code (Example: 66984 (ECCE/IOL)—55)
Evaluation and management service unrelated to surgery	Modifier 24 preceded by evaluation/management code (see below) (Example: 99214 (office visit, detailed)—24)
Procedure or surgical service unrelated to surgery	Modifier 79 preceded by procedure code (Example: 65222 (foreign body removal)—79)
Postoperative visits 90 days or more after surgery	
Eye codes	
Established patient—comprehensive	92014
Established patient—intermediate	92012
Evaluation/management medical codes	
Office visit—problem focused	99212
Office visit—expanded	99213
Office visit—detailed	99214
Procedure codes	
Visual fields, photos, and other tests as indicated	Appropriate procedure code (see Table 7.1.)
Refraction	92015*
Fitting for spectacle lenses	92352
Frames	V2020
Lens (material)	V code RT/LT
Fitting monocular contact lens	92311
Contact lens (material)	V code RT/LT

*Refraction should be billed. It will be denied as a noncovered service by Medicare, and the provider can then collect the fee from the patient.

Table 7.3 CPT Codes Used in the Postoperative Cataract Evaluation

Diagnosis	ICD-9 Code
Cataract (unspecified type)	366.9
Anterior subcapsular	366.13
Congenital	743.30
Cortical	366.15
Drug-induced	366.45
Juvenile	366.00
Nuclear sclerosis	366.16
Posterior subcapsular	366.14
Pseudoexfoliation of lens capsule	366.11
Traumatic	366.20
After cataract (opacified capsule)	366.50
Aphakia	379.31
Pseudophakia	V43.1

Table 7.4   Selected ICD-9 Diagnostic Codes Used in the Pre- and Postoperative Cataract Evaluation

□ Medicare

Medicare is a federally subsidized health insurance program for the elderly (over age 65) and disabled, established by Congress in 1965 as part of the Social Security system. Medicare falls under the jurisdiction of the HCFA, a division of the U.S. Department of Health and Human Services (HHS). Optometrists have been included in the Medicare program since 1987. Under the Medicare system, postoperative care provided by the surgeon is included in the surgical fee. This is termed the *global fee*. When postoperative care is provided by a doctor of optometry, the global fee is broken down into surgical and postoperative care components as follows:

The surgeon uses *modifier 54* (surgical care only) when the majority of the postoperative care is delivered by another practitioner. This modifier is used along with the surgical procedure code. For example,

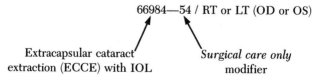

66984—54 / RT or LT (OD or OS)

Extracapsular cataract extraction (ECCE) with IOL

Surgical care only modifier

Filed by surgeon

The use of this modifier alerts Medicare to reduce reimbursement to the surgeon by 20 percent. This amount is then used to pay the optometrist for follow-up care provided within ninety days of the surgery.

In order to be reimbursed, the optometrist should file the appropriate surgical code followed by *modifier 55*, indicating postoperative co-management with an ophthalmic surgeon. For example:

66984—55 / RT or LT

ECCE with IOL   *Postoperative care* modifier

Filed by optometrist

While the usual number of follow-up visits for a routine surgery is three or four, any additional visits are included in the global fee and cannot be billed separately. Surgical or medical services provided during the postoperative period that are *unrelated to the surgery* may be billed using the appropriate modifier—*modifier 24* for medical services and *modifier 79* for surgical services—and will be approved at the full fee schedule amount. For example:

65222—79

Corneal Foreign Body Removal   Surgical Modifier for Procedure Done
during 90 day Postoperative Period,
unrelated to the surgery.

After 90 days, billing for individual office visits and diagnostic tests can resume as before surgery. Always consult with the individual carrier on how to bill for co-managed cataract care as the general guidelines listed above can vary slightly from state to state.

The only time Medicare pays for eye wear is following cataract surgery. For pseudophakes, coverage will be provided for only one pair of glasses per cataract surgery per lifetime. Coverage is also allowed for a contact lens and reading glasses in place of conventional bifocals. Pseudophakic prescription changes and lost or broken eye wear are not covered by Medicare. The provider, of course, can bill the patient for these noncovered services. Aphakes, on the other hand, are allowed coverage for corrective lenses each time the prescription changes.

RESOURCE-BASED RELATIVE VALUE SCALE (RBRVS)

Medicare payment for physician services has been dramatically affected by reforms implemented in January of 1992. The new fee schedule represents the most significant change in physician reimbursement since the inception of the Medicare program. The fees are based on the relative values of doctors' work, overhead, and malpractice expenses, not on "prevailing and reasonable charges" as in the past. The system is intended to reduce historically large payments to specialists such as ophthalmologists and anesthesiologists and to increase fees paid to primary-care doctors such as optometrists and general practitioners (Figure 7.4). The goal is not to reduce total spending but rather to redistribute the money in an effort to encourage more doctors to enter primary care. The new fee schedule may have implications beyond the Medicare program. Private insurance companies are evaluating these new fees as a possible guide in determining how much to pay doctors in the future.

CATARACT DEMONSTRATION PROJECT

Cataract surgery represents a significant percentage of the Medicare budget—by some estimates at least $2.5 billion annually. In an effort to provide incentives to physicians to keep costs down, the *Medicare Cataract Surgery Alternate Payment Demonstration* is under way. By negotiating a *package price* of fees related to cataract surgery, HCFA is hoping to motivate surgical providers to control surgical and facility costs carefully.

Providers in several cities will participate in this three-year study. The project will then be analyzed in terms of efficiency and savings to the Medicare system. The model is based on a *bundled fee*, which includes:

Preoperative Care	Surgical Care	Postoperative Care
Presurgical exam and diagnostic tests 7-day waiting period	Surgeon Anesthesiologist Facility IOL	Postoperative exams (approximately 4) Final refraction and glasses

Rather than paying for each service separately, Medicare will *bundle* the fees and pay the surgeon a lump sum. The anesthesiology, surgery, facility, and postoperative fees are paid from this bundled fee. This places the burden on the physician and facility to do each case as cost effectively as possible. Medicare will pay less for the *package* than it would for each service separately and therefore cut costs. Providers not participating in the demonstration project will be paid in the conventional way.

☐ Medicaid

Medicaid is a joint federal and state health-care program for qualified low-income patients. Reimbursement for postoperative care delivered by optometrists to Medicaid patients varies from state to state. Medicaid does not recognize the global fee in some states but does in others. Local carrier-assigned codes and coverage information can be obtained from local Medicaid offices.

Change by Specialty		
Percentage gain or loss relative to the national average in payments per service.		
Physician	1992	1996
Family practice	+16%	+37%
General practice	+18	+36
Cardiology	-3%	-1%
Gastroenterology	-4	+10
Neurology	-1	+8
Pulmonary	-1	+9
Radiology	-3%	-19%
Anesthesiology	-5	-22
Pathology	-4	-17
General surgery	-2%	-5%
Neurosurgery	-4	-10
Ophthalmology	**-6**	**-22**
Orthopedic surgery	-4	-3
Clinics	+2%	+7%
Optometry	**+16**	**+33**
Podiatry	+8	+39

Change by Service			

Medicare payments for physician services under the current system and under the new fee schedule. The samples below, from a list of more than 4,000 services, are in current dollars; the fees in 1992 and 1996 will be adjusted for inflation in physicians' costs.

Service	1991	1992	1996
Chest X-ray	$ 14	$ 13	$ 9
Typical hospital visit	30	36	38
Typical office visit	38	45	48
Contrast CAT scans, abdomen	91	82	57
Weekly radiation therapy	162	147	99
Repair inguinal hernia	439	395	292
Inserting heart pacemaker	818	744	491
Gallbladder removal	746	683	525
Total hysterectomy	837	748	592
Removing cataract, inserting lens	**1,342**	**1,210**	**832**
Total hip joint replacement	2,111	1,888	1,486
Coronary artery bypass	3,181	2,892	1,925

Figure 7.4 The RBRVS Medicare fee schedule, showing increases and cuts in reimbursement based on specialty and service. (Courtesy Department of Health and Human Services.)

□ Private Insurance

Private insurance carriers usually do not recognize the breaking out of the global fee into surgical and postoperative components and thus do not presently pay optometrists for postoperative care. Until they do, bill each visit separately as a medical follow-up with a diagnosis of aphakia. Some insurance carriers will reimburse for these visits. Appeals made to individual carriers on a case-by-case basis will hopefully result in routine reimbursement of postoperative care in the future.

Suggested Reading

Adamsons I et al. Prevalence of lens opacities in surgical and general populations. *Arch Ophthalmol* 1991; 109:993–997.

Assia E, Apple D. An experimental study comparing various capsulectomy techniques. *Arch Ophthalmol* 1991; 109:642–647.

Assia E et al. Mechanism of radial tear formation and extension after anterior capsulectomy. *Ophthalmology* 1991; 98:432–437.

Barresi B. Ocular assessment. Boston: Butterworth–Heinemann, 1984.

Battelle Human Affairs Research Centers. Outcomes of cataract surgery with co-managed postoperative care. Washington, D.C.: Battelle Human Affairs Research Centers, 1990.

Bradley, D. Medicare reimbursement workshop manual. Atlanta: Omni Eye Services, 1990.

Brazitikos, P, Roth A. Iris modifications following extracapsular cataract extraction with posterior chamber lens implantation. *J Cataract Refract Surg* 1991; 17:269–280.

Brint S, Ostrick M. The evolution of small-incision cataract surgery with foldable IOL's. *J Am Optom Assoc* 1991; 62:365–371.

Cionni R, Osher R. Retrobulbar hemorrhage. *Opththalmology* 1991; 98:1153–1155.

Classé J. Legal aspects of optometry. Boston: Butterworth–Heinemann, 1989.

Classé J, ed. *Optometry Clinics*, 1991; 1(2).

Driebe WT, Mandlebaum S, Forster RK, et al. Pseudophakic endophthalmitis. *Ophthalmology* 1986; 93:442.

Eskridge B, Amos J, Bartlett J. Clinical procedures in optometry. Philadelphia: Lippincott, 1991.

Fingeret M, Casser L, Woodcome T. Atlas of primary eyecare procedures. Norwalk, Conn.: Appleton & Lange, 1991.

Garston M. Co-management of the cataract/pseudophakic patient. *Contact Lens Spectrum* May 1991; 28–40.

Gimbel H, Sanders D, Raanan M. Visual and refractive results of multifocal intraocular lenses. *Ophthalmology* 1991; 98:881–888.

Glasser D et al. Endothelial protection and viscoelastic retention during phacoemulsification and intraocular lens implantation. *Arch Ophthalmol* 1991; 109:1438–1440.

Gutner R. Pseudoexfoliation syndrome. *Clin Eye & Vision Care* 1988; 1:48–49.

Hamed L. Strabismus presenting after cataract surgery. *Ophthalmology* 1991; 98:247–252.

Hattenhauer J. To "phaco" or not. *Arch Ophthalmol* 1991; 109:315.

Hay A et al. Needle penetration of the globe during retrobulbar and peribulbar injections. *Ophthalmology* 1991; 98:1017–1023.

Isaac N et al. Exposure to phenothiazine drugs and risk of cataract. *Arch Ophthalmol* 1991; 109:256–260.

Jaffe N, Jaffe M, Jaffe G. Cataract surgery and its complications. St. Louis: Mosby, 1990.

Kanski J. Clinical ophthalmology. London: Butterworth–Heinemann, 1989.

Lane S et al. Prospective comparison of the effects of Occucoat, Viscoat, and Healon on intraocular pressure and endothelial cell loss. *J Cataract Refract Surg* 1991; 17:21–26.

Leske, C et al. The lens opacities case control study: Risk factors for cataract. *Arch Ophthalmol* 1991; 109:244–251.

Lindquist T, Lindstrom R. Ophthalmic surgery. Chicago: Year Book Medical Publishers, 1990.

March W. Ophthalmology Clinics of North America. *Practical Laser Surgery* 1989; 2(4).

Milaushas A. Silicone intraocular lens implant discoloration in humans. *Arch Ophthalmol* 1991; 109:913.

Moisseiev J et al. Long-term study of the prevalence of capsular opacification following extracapsular cataract extraction. *J Cataract Refract Surg* 1989; 15:531–533.

Montalto S. Lovostatin and cataracts: An update. *Clin Eye & Vision Care*, 1989; 1:212–217.

Moses, R. Adler's Physiology of the Eye. St. Louis: Mosby, 1975.

Quinn, C. Cataract management: An optometric guide. Iselin, N.J.: C Quinn 1989.

Records, R. Physiology of the eye and human visual system. Hagerstown, Md.: Harper & Row, 1979.

Rivicki D, Brown R, Adler M. Outcomes of cataract surgery with co-managed postoperative care. Washington D.C.; Battelle Human Affairs Research Center, 1989.

Steele A, Drews R. Cataract surgery. London: Butterworth–Heinemann, 1984.

Steinert R et al. Astigmatism after small incision cataract surgery: A prospective, randomized, multicenter comparison of 4 and 6.5mm incisions. *Ophthalmology* 1991; 98:417–424.

Tasman W, Jaeger E. Duane's Clinical Ophthalmology, vol 1. Philadelphia: Lippincott, 1990.

Whitmer L. Trends in IOL's: Design, surgery, complications. *Southern Journal of Optometry* 1989; 8:39–44.

Zahl K, Meltzer M. Ophthalmology clinics of North America. *Regional anesthesia for intraocular surgery* 1990; 3(1).

Index